THE EVALUATOR'S GUIDE *TO ACCOMPANY*
MOSBY'S CLINICAL DECISION AND COMPETENCY EVALUATION VIDEO SERIES FOR RESPIRATORY CARE

THE EVALUATOR'S GUIDE *TO ACCOMPANY* MOSBY'S CLINICAL DECISION AND COMPETENCY EVALUATION VIDEO SERIES FOR RESPIRATORY CARE

Patricia Fuchs Carroll, MS, RRT, RN
Owner
Educational Medical Consultants
Middletown, Connecticut
Adjunct Faculty, Respiratory Care
Manchester Community-Technical College
Manchester, Connecticut

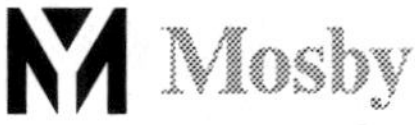

St. Louis Baltimore Boston Carlsbad Chicago Naples New York Philadelphia Portland
London Madrid Mexico City Singapore Sydney Tokyo Toronto Wiesbaden

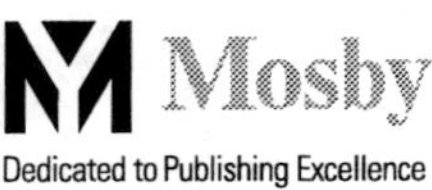

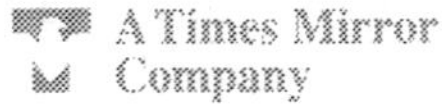

Publisher: Don Ladig
Editor: Jennifer Roche
Developmental Editor: Anne Gleason
Project Manager: Gayle Morris
Production Editor: Gina Keckritz
Layout Artist: Ken Wendling
Designer: Guy Jacobs

Printed in the United States of America
Composition by Wordbench

Mosby-Year Book, Inc.
11830 Westline Industrial Drive
St. Louis, Missouri 63146

ISBN:0-8151-1475-3

96 97 98 99 00 / 9 8 7 6 5 4 3 2 1

Table of Contents

INTRODUCTION
How to Use the Clinical Decision Series 1
How to Use the Competency Evaluation Series 4
Tips for Teaching with Videos 5

PART 1 - CLINICAL DECISION SERIES

Introductory Unit Introduction to Clinical Decision Making
Learning Objectives 9
Video Outline 9
References 11

Unit 1 Oxygen Therapy
Learning Objectives 13
Video Outline 14
Video Assessment Findings 15
Suggested Teaching Points 16
Student Workbook Topics 16
References 16

Unit 2 Aerosol Therapy
Learning Objectives 19
Video Outline 20
Video Assessment Findings 21
Suggested Teaching Points 22
Student Workbook Topics 22
References 22

Unit 3 Secretion Management
Learning Objectives 25
Video Outline 26
Video Assessment Findings 27
Suggested Teaching Points 28
Student Workbook Topics 29
References 29

Unit 4 Volume Expansion
Learning Objectives 31
Video Outline 32
Video Assessment Findings 33
Suggested Teaching Points 34
Student Workbook Topics 35
References 35

Unit 5 Physical Assessment
Learning Objectives 37
Video Outline 38
Video Assessment Findings 39
Suggested Teaching Points 40
Student Workbook Topics 41
References 41

Unit 6 Pediatrics
Learning Objectives 43
Video Outline 44
Video Assessment Findings 45
Suggested Teaching Points 46
Student Workbook Topics 46
References 46

Unit 7 Noninvasive Monitoring
Learning Objectives 49
Video Outline 50
Video Assessment Findings 52
Suggested Teaching Points 52
Student Workbook Topics 53
References 53

Unit 8 Mechanical Ventilation
Learning Objectives 55
Video Outline 56
Video Assessment Findings 58
Suggested Teaching Points 59
Student Workbook Topics 59
References 60

PART II - THE COMPETENCY EVALUATION SERIES

Competency Evaluation Questions and Suggested Responses

Unit 1 Oxygen Therapy
Question Set 1 63
Question Set 2 63
Question Set 3 64
Question Set 4 65

Unit 2 Aerosol Therapy
Question Set 1 67
Question Set 2 67
Question Set 3 68
Question Set 4 69

Unit 3 Secretion Management
Question Set 1 71
Question Set 2 71
Question Set 3 72
Question Set 4 73

Unit 4 Volume Expansion
Question Set 1 75
Question Set 2 75
Question Set 3 76
Question Set 4 77

Unit 5 Physical Assessment
Question Set 1 79
Question Set 2 79
Question Set 3 81

Unit 6 Pediatrics
Question Set 1 83
Question Set 2 83
Question Set 3 84
Question Set 4 84
Question Set 5 85

Unit 7 Noninvasive Monitoring
Question Set 1 87
Question Set 2 87
Question Set 3 88
Question Set 4 88

Unit 8 Mechanical Ventilation
Question Set 1 89
Question Set 2 89
Question Set 3 89
Question Set 4 90
Question Set 5 90

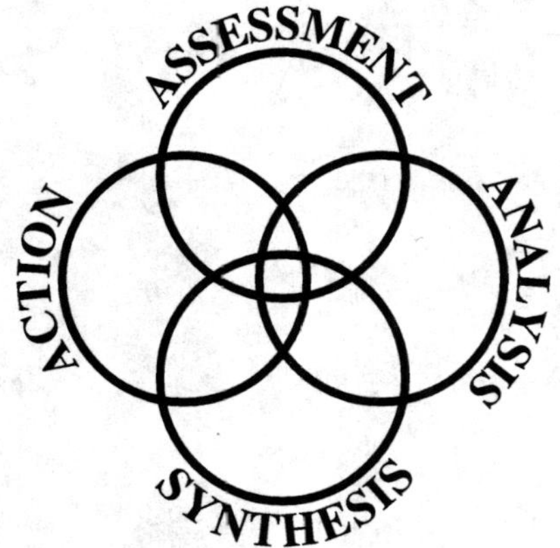

Introduction

How to Use the Clinical Decision Series

This series is designed to help teach and develop clinical decision making skills in respiratory care students and practitioners. This series is composed of eight case study videos, an introductory video, and a companion student workbook. Each video addresses a separate skill area in the context of a case study of a patient with a specific disease or condition:

Oxygen Therapy	COPD
Aerosol Therapy	Asthma
Secretion Management	Pneumonia
Volume Expansion	Postoperative Abdominal Aortic Aneurysm
Physical Assessment	Chest Trauma with Pneumothorax
Pediatrics	Croup
Noninvasive Monitoring	Tricyclic Antidepressant Overdose
Mechanical Ventilation	Myocardial Infarction with Heart Failure and Pulmonary Edema

There are two video sets: the *Clinical Decision Series* and the *Competency Evaluation Series*. Videos in the *Clinical Decision Series* follow four phases of the **clinical decision-making model** through clinical case-study footage and expert commentary:

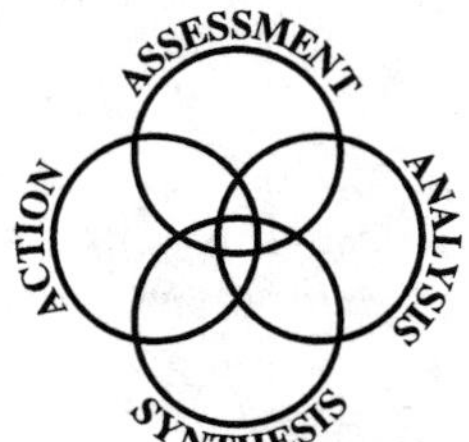

Assessment, in which the viewer collects subjective and objective data about the patient;
Analysis, in which the viewer reviews the pathophysiology relating to the assessment data;
Synthesis, where the viewer applies the assessment data and pathophysiology to a protocol for care; and
Action, the segment in which therapy is administered and results are evaluated

The video *Introduction to Clinical Decision Making* describes these steps in greater detail.

The videos combine clinical case study scenes with expert commentary. The clinical scenes are shot from a "you-are-there" perspective to provide the most realistic clinical simulation possible. The patient interview is conducted from the viewer/RCP's actual point of view; viewers hear heart and breath sounds through the stethoscope as if they were conducting the examination themselves. Because of this unique perspective, we do not use graphics to point out clinical findings; we let the clinical footage stand on its own to provide you with maximum instructional flexibility.

A companion video series, the *Competency Evaluation Series*, provides the clinical scenes alone. These videos are designed for assessment of senior-level students and practitioners. Please see "How to Use the Competency Evaluation Series" in this Evaluator's Guide for additional information.

EVALUATOR'S GUIDE

Part One of this Evaluator's Guide provides the instructor with comprehensive support materials for each clinical case video to facilitate curriculum integration.

Learning Objectives. A set of learning objectives is provided for each case. Objectives address the cognitive domain, according to Bloom's taxonomy. This taxonomy is organized into two major groups: simple recall of information and higher intellectual activities. Content in each case study video provides information applicable to each domain. This allows you to use the series in both technician and therapist programs and for both novice and more experienced students and practitioners. The key to this instructional flexibility is the application activities you facilitate in the classroom before and after the video is shown. You may decide to use the objectives as a guide to developing complimentary classroom activities and assignments.

Video Outline. A detailed content outline is provided for each case. This makes it easier for you to preview the content covered in each case and to focus on key areas that link these cases to your curriculum.

Assessment Findings Presented in Video. We understand that there will be great variations in the equipment available for presenting these videos in the classroom. In some cases, the use of small-screen television monitors may make words on the screen difficult to read. To address this potential problem, this section provides you with a summary of the clinical findings so you can present them to students yourself if necessary. In addition, this summary provides you with additional information as you preview the video's content for curriculum integration.

Suggested Teaching Points. As instructional designers, we feel very strongly that videos are a tool to compliment the instructor, not replace the instructor. Please see "How to Teach with Videos" for more tips on using this media tool. To assist you with follow-up activities to supplement the use of these videos in class, these suggestions are provided as a starting point for classroom discussion and related activities. They are by no means exhaustive, and we encourage you to build on these suggestions with particular attention to customizing your activities based on the needs of and resources available at your school and clinical affiliate(s). Use these suggestions to develop instructional strategies as an alternative to the traditional lecture. A list of student workbook topics is also included in this section to help you plan student assignments at various points in your curriculum.

References. A list of the sources used to write the video scripts is included for each case to supplement your classroom activities. A fully integrated bibliography is included in the student workbook.

CURRICULUM INTEGRATION

Each of the videos can be used at various points in your curriculum. Don't hesitate to use only parts of the video (chosen with the assistance of the outline) or to use a video more than once to emphasize different content—or to have the student focus on a different aspect of the case. Each case begins with a patient assessment; these segments can also be used alone when teaching physical assessment skills.

Other curriculum integration options:

Oxygen Therapy
- Physical assessment
- Respiratory physiology: types of hypoxia
- Respiratory diseases: COPD
- Equipment: oxygen administration devices
- Procedures: oxygen administration
- Critical thinking: TDP for oxygen therapy

Aerosol Therapy
- Physical assessment
- Respiratory diseases: asthma
- Equipment: aerosol delivery devices
- Procedures: SVN administration with assessment of results
- Critical thinking: TDP for choosing aerosol delivery device

Secretion Management
- Physical assessment
- Respiratory physiology: mucociliary clearance
- Respiratory diseases: pneumonia
- Procedures: CPT/PD
- Critical thinking: TDP for bronchial hygiene

Volume Expansion
- Physical assessment
- Respiratory physiology: normal respiratory changes with aging
- Respiratory diseases: atelectasis, postoperative risk
- Equipment: incentive spirometry, IPPB

Procedures: incentive spirometry
Critical thinking: TDP for choosing volume expansion device

Physical Assessment/Chest Trauma

Physical assessment: in depth
Respiratory physiology: oxygen-carrying capacity
Respiratory diseases: chest trauma, pneumothorax
Equipment: nonrebreather mask, chest drainage
Critical thinking: trauma primary assessment and intervention protocol

Pediatrics

Physical assessment
Respiratory physiology: changes in pediatric airway compared to adult airway
Respiratory diseases: croup and epiglottitis
Equipment: SVN
Critical thinking: administering therapy to children

Noninvasive Monitoring

Physical assessment
Respiratory diseases: drug overdose
Equipment: EKG monitoring, pulse oximetry, capnography
Critical thinking: TDP for pulse oximetry, indications for each device

Mechanical Ventilation

Physical assessment
Respiratory disease: cardiogenic pulmonary edema
Equipment: mechanical ventilator, PEEP
Critical thinking: TDP for mechanical ventilation, applying pathophysiology

Videos can be used to introduce topics or to summarize after the unit is taught. Individual videos can be used in the students' first year for basic information and then introduced later in the curriculum to teach the integration and application of knowledge necessary to develop clinical decision making skills.

STUDENT WORKBOOK

Similarly, the student workbook can be integrated into your entire curriculum as well. Each student should have his or her own workbook. Specific workbook topics are listed after "Suggested Teaching Points" for each video in this Evaluator's Guide. The questions are related to the content in each video, but the student does not have to watch the entire video in order to answer the questions. Resources that were used to develop the questions and answers are noted in the workbook to help direct the student, but these particular resources are not required. We encourage students to use any resources available to them, including books from other disciplines such as medicine and nursing, as well as professional resources. Workbook questions also address different cognitive levels; some questions require more work and research by the student than others. A multiple-question posttest summarizes each unit. We strongly recommend discussion of answers to questions in class to help clarify and reinforce content rather than simply assigning work for self-study. Answers to questions in the workbook are developed from the resources cited at the start of each workbook unit. If other resources are used, student responses may differ slightly. This can best be addressed through classroom discussion of the nuances of the topic.

The therapist-driven protocols used in the series are reprinted in the workbook. We suggest you point this out so students can follow along when the protocol is discussed in the video.

How to Use the Competency Evaluation Series

This series is designed to help you assess clinical decision making skills in respiratory care students and practitioners. This series is composed of eight case study videos, an introductory video, and a companion workbook. Each video addresses a separate skill area in the context of a case study of a patient with a specific disease or condition:

Oxygen Therapy	COPD
Aerosol Therapy	Asthma
Secretion Management	Pneumonia
Volume Expansion	Postoperative Abdominal Aortic Aneurysm
Physical Assessment	Chest Trauma with Pneumothorax
Pediatrics	Croup
Noninvasive Monitoring	Tricyclic Antidepressant Overdose
Mechanical Ventilation	Myocardial Infarction with Heart Failure and Pulmonary Edema

There are two video sets: the *Clinical Decision Series* and the *Competency Evaluation Series*. Videos in the *Clinical Decision Series* follow four phases of the **clinical decision-making model** through clinical case study footage and expert commentary. The *Competency Evaluation Series* provides the clinical footage alone. At logical places in the case, the video stops and the viewer is directed to answer workbook questions. Each viewer should have his or her own workbook in which to answer the competency assessment questions.

JCAHO AND COMPETENCY ASSESSMENT

In 1995, the Joint Commission on Accreditation of Healthcare Organizations (JCAHO) began surveying hospitals under the revised *Accreditation Manual*. A key element of this revision is the aspect of human resource management. Surveyors are looking at how competence relates to orientation, continuing education, and annual evaluation. Many institutions have done an excellent job assessing psychomotor skills through the use of checklists. These task-oriented tools focus on setting up equipment properly and troubleshooting problems. Newly hired staff can be evaluated with these checklists to assess entry-level skills and identify areas requiring remediation. Staff members can be evaluated on a regular basis.

A common dilemma for managers of respiratory care services is developing a method for assessing and evaluating cognitive or clinical decision making skills. This series was designed by registered respiratory therapists to meet this need. Newly hired staff can be assigned all eight cases. Designated management personnel can review the responses, along with other assessment data, such as psychomotor checklists, to develop a customized orientation plan for each new hire. By customizing orientation, the process can often be shortened, making it more cost effective.

Staff members can be assessed annually, choosing cases at random or on a rotating schedule. An analysis of staff members' responses to the cases can form the basis for department-wide continuing and inservice education to remediate common areas of substandard performance. This strategy will enhance department-wide competence and can be monitored with established departmental quality indicators. Remediation can be accomplished with the companion Clinical Decision video series. Please see the "How to Use the Clinical Decision Series" in this evaluator's guide for additional information.

JCAHO also requires competency in administering therapy across the lifespan. This series also helps address that requirement. The Pediatric video addresses needs of children of various ages, and the Volume Expansion video discusses normal changes associated with aging in the setting of a postoperative patient. This series addresses pediatric, adult, and geriatric patient populations.

New standards also require surveyors to assess how respiratory care departments meet standards for patient assessment. Each video in this series begins with a patient assessment, and the workbook questions require interpretation of assessment findings.

Each video addresses patient education for various treatment modalities, and the Physical Assessment, Noninvasive Monitoring, and Mechanical Ventilation videos highlight collaborative practice between RCPs and registered nurses. These are additional areas of special interest to the JCAHO.

IMPLEMENTING COMPETENCY ASSESSMENT WITH THE VIDEO SERIES

The *Workbook To Accompany the Clinical Decision Video Series* can be used for intensive study and review in specific content areas. The *Workbook To Accompany the Competency Evaluation Video Series* is designed for assessment of the senior level respiratory student and practicing professional. Suggested responses to the questions for the *Competency Evaluation* workbook are provided in this Evaluator's Guide. Responses are written on the basis of national standards; notations are made when specific responses depend on individual institutional polices and procedures. In any case, the suggested responses are only that—suggested. Designated department management personnel should review the suggested responses and modify them as needed to customize them for the institution. Therapist-driven protocols (TDPs) used in the videos are included as an appendix in the workbooks. If your institution uses TDPs, you can substitute your own.

The *Competency Evaluation* workbook is perforated so that each case can be presented as a test of competency in that subject area. The student's responses can then be documented and put on file to prove competency. This unique approach to competency assessment can be performed at any time. For example, the videotape, questions, and video equipment can be left for night-shift employees to complete on their own; management personnel do not necessarily need to be present.

Responses should be analyzed in two ways: individual responses should be reviewed and discussed with individual RCPs and remediation assigned as necessary. Department-wide responses should be assessed in aggregate to determine if common errors are made. These common areas should then be addressed with department-wide continuing or in-service educaton. The *Clinical Decision Series* videos and workbook can be used for this purpose.

Tips for Teaching with Videos

Using video as one element of multimedia instructional support is an art. The success of this approach lies partly in the quality of the video itself and partly in the plans the instructor uses to integrate the video into the curriculum. Here are some tips to the successful use of video, along with questions to consider.

- ❑ Think about your viewers. Are they content novices or experts? What is their previous experience with video instruction? How will that affect the experience you're planning? What will you need to do to prepare them?

- ❑ Develop specific objectives. In addition to content objectives, set objectives for the use of video. Why are you using this medium? What do you expect to accomplish? Focus on these important objectives. Keep them specific, measurable, and attainable.

- ❑ Preview the video. You should be familiar with the content and how the video presents that content. Write notes about points made in the video that you want to emphasize or reinforce.

- ❑ Don't hesitate to stop the video in order to point out important points—or to rewind it to show them a second time. (Hopefully, you made notes of these points when you previewed the video.) Stop the video and ask questions of the viewers—what would they do next?

- ❑ Require performance from the viewer. The best plans for video use can fall apart if this step is omitted. It is critical that the viewer be directed to apply information presented in the video. It can be as simple as a worksheet the viewer completes while watching—or as sophisticated as the workbook exercises that accompany this video series. Follow-up discussions and activities, provided in the "Suggested Teaching Points" sections of this evaluator's guide, also require viewer performance. Proper instructional management of this step is an art and will greatly enhance content retention.

- ❑ Most of all, have fun with the process. Experiment and try different approaches. Some will work better than others. Make the most of your resources and share your experiences with your colleagues.

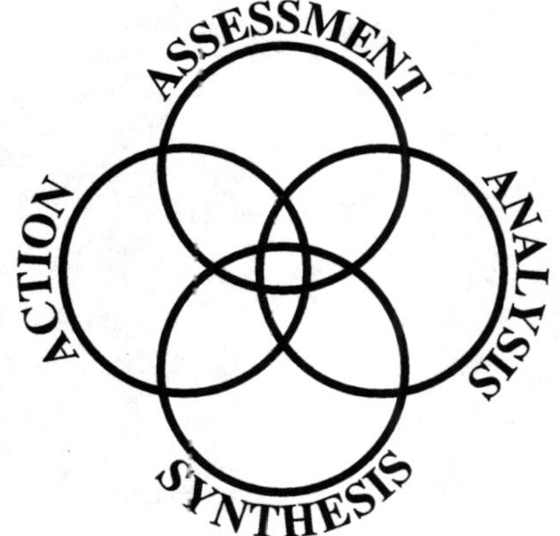

Part I

Clinical Decision Series

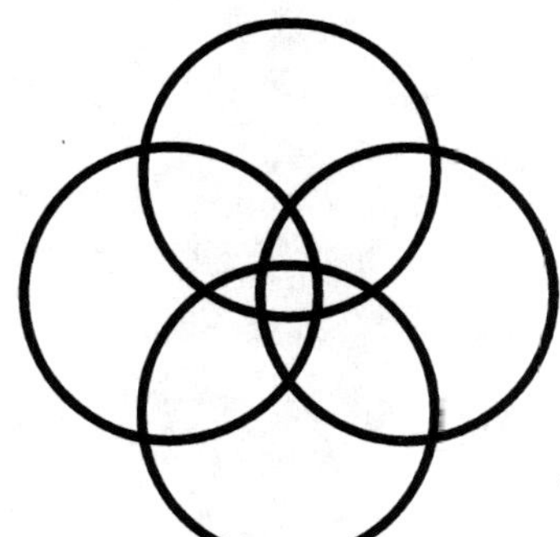

Introduction to Clinical Decision Making

Learning Objectives

At the end of this program, the learner should be able to...

Knowledge

...list the four components of a chest physical exam.
...name four components of the Clinical Decision-Making Model described in the video.

Comprehension

...describe the use of AARC Clinical Practice Guidelines.
...contrast clinical signs and clinical symptoms.

Application

...classify a given piece of patient assessment data as a sign or symptom.
...choose the appropriate TDP for a given patient.

Analysis

...compare and contrast the data available from inspection, palpation, percussion, and auscultation.
...diagram the Clinical Decision-Making Model discussed in the video, showing relationships between the four elements of the model.

Synthesis

...summarize the four steps of the Clinical Decision-Making Model discussed in the video.
...explain why it is so important to apply knowledge of pathophysiology to TDPs.

Evaluation

Because this is an introductory video, this cognitive level is not addressed.

Video Outline

I. Introduction
    A. Credentialling exam pass rates
    B. Therapist-driven protocols
    C. Importance of expert clinical decision making skills
II. Clinical Decision-Making Model
    A. Four steps
        1. Assessment
        2. Analysis
        3. Synthesis

4. Action

III. Assessment
   A. Subjective data
      1. Data evident to the patient
      2. Patient's perception
      3. Symptoms
   B. Objective data
      1. Data seen, felt, heard, or smelled by RCP
      2. Clinical signs
   C. Interview
      1. Chief complaint
      2. History of present illness
      3. Past medical history
   D. Physical examination
      1. Inspection
         a. Breathing pattern, effort, configuration of chest, scars
      2. Palpation
         a. Skin temperature, hydration, diaphoresis
         b. Tactile fremitus
         c. Bony injuries (trauma patients)
      3. Percussion
         a. Resonance
      4. Auscultation
         a. Clinical examples
            (1) Tubular/bronchial
            (2) Decreased aeration
            (3) Wheezes
            (4) Stridor
      5. Other techniques
         a. Capillary refill
         b. Peripheral edema
         c. Noninvasive monitoring
   E. Review chart
      1. Laboratory, x-ray, notes

IV. Analysis
   A. Pathophysiology
      1. Hypoxia
         a. Four types
      2. Pneumonia
      3. Pneumothorax
      4. CHF/pulmonary edema
   B. Discussion
      1. Treating pathophysiology, not just symptoms

V. Synthesis
   A. Therapist-driven protocols
      1. Definition
      2. Review of protocol for bronchodilator therapy
         a. Critical thinking analysis
         b. Follows protocol
      3. Review of protocol for mechanical ventilation
         a. Critical thinking analysis
         b. Does not follow protocol exactly

c. Application of pathophysiology
B. Goals for therapy
1. Development of goals
a. SMART: specific, measurable, attainable, realistic, time-frame
2. Oxygen therapy as example
a. Analysis of goals
VI. Action
A. Administering therapy
1. AARC Clinical Practice Guidelines
a. Definition
b. Application
VII. Summary

References

Hess D: The AARC clinical practice guidelines, Resp Care 36:1398-1401, 1991.

Jacobs J: How are we doing with operational restructuring and therapist-driven protocols? In AARC Times 18:66-69, 1994.

National Board for Respiratory Care: NBRC '94 examination statistics, NBRC Horizons, March-April: 6-7, 1995.

Weber K and Milligan S: Therapist-driven protocols: the state of the art, Resp Care 39:746-756, 1994.

Wilkins RL, Krider SJ, and Sheldon RL, editors: Clinical assessment in respiratory care, ed 3, St. Louis, 1995, Mosby.

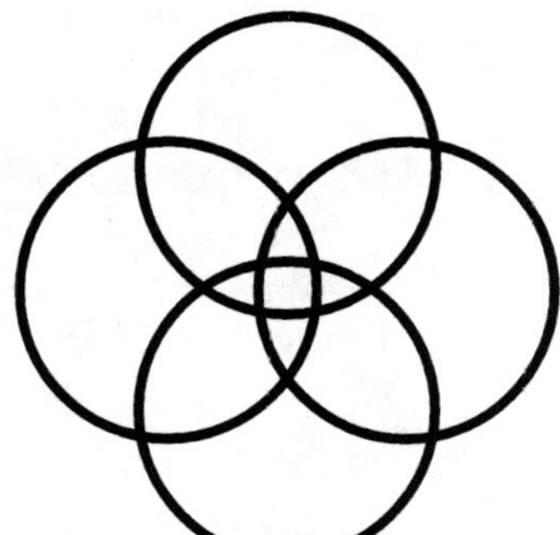

Oxygen Therapy

Learning Objectives

At the end of this program, the learner should be able to...

Knowledge

...list four types of hypoxia.
...define hypoxemic hypoxia, anemic hypoxia, circulatory hypoxia, and histotoxic hypoxia.
...recognize assessment findings that indicate hypoxia in Mr. Feder.

Comprehension

...describe Mr. Feder's breath sounds.
...summarize Mr. Feder's chief complaint, history of present illness, and past medical history.
...contrast the four types of hypoxia.

Application

...apply Mr. Feder's assessment findings to an oxygen therapy protocol.
...classify Mr. Feder's type of hypoxia.
...write goals for oxygen therapy for Mr. Feder.

Analysis

...compare and contrast the four types of hypoxia.
...separate relevant from irrelevant findings in Mr. Feder's history and physical assessment.
...analyze Mr. Feder's response to therapy.

Synthesis

...integrate Mr. Feder's assessment findings with the types of hypoxia.
...formulate a plan of care for Mr. Feder, based on assessment findings.
...develop a teaching plan for Mr. Feder.

Evaluation

...evaluate the results of interventions for Mr. Feder.
...reassess the appropriateness of Mr. Feder's care plan.
...recommend the next step in Mr. Feder's respiratory care.

Video Outline

- I. Introduction
  - A. History of oxygen therapy
- II. Assessment
  - A. Referral from nurse
    - 1. Vital signs
  - B. RCP interview
    - 1. Chief complaint
    - 2. History of present illness
    - 3. Past medical history
  - C. Physical examination
    - 1. Pulse oximetry
    - 2. Inspection
    - 3. Palpation
    - 4. Percussion
    - 5. Auscultation
  - D. Discussion
    - 1. Tripod position
    - 2. Pursed-lip breathing
    - 3. Potential causes of hypoxemia
      - a. Cardiac
      - b. Acute infection
    - 4. Numerical dyspnea scale
    - 5. Mental status
- III. Analysis
  - A. Types of hypoxia
    - 1. Hypoxemic hypoxia
      - a. Definition
      - b. Causes of low PaO_2
        - (1) Low alveolar oxygen
        - (2) Impaired diffusion
        - (3) Right-to-left shunt
        - (4) $\dot{V}/\dot{Q}$ mismatch
    - 2. Anemic hypoxia
      - a. Definition
    - 3. Circulatory hypoxia
      - a. Definition
        - (1) Circulatory failure/shock
        - (2) Ischemia
    - 4. Histotoxic hypoxia
      - a. Definition
  - B. Mr. Feder's findings applied to types of hypoxia
    - 1. Hypoxemic hypoxia
- IV. Synthesis
  - A. Therapist-driven protocol for oxygen therapy
    - 1. Mr. Feder's findings applied to the protocol
    - 2. Nasal cannula
  - B. Goals of therapy
    - 1. Improve oxygenation
    - 2. Decrease dyspnea

3. Reduce cardiac workload

V. Action
   A. Applying nasal cannula
   B. Patient teaching
   C. Reassessment
      1. Lab values
      2. Patient assessment

VI. Summary
   A. Oxygen as drug
   B. Indications for oxygen therapy
      1. Hypoxemia/hypoxia
      2. Compensatory mechanisms
      3. Decrease work of breathing
      4. Balance myocardial oxygen supply and demand
   C. Harmful effects
      1. Oxygen therapy
      2. Hypoventilation
      3. Absorption atelectasis
      4. Retinopathy of prematurity

Video Assessment Findings

Initial nursing assessment:

RR 24, HR 104, BP 144/82, T 99 tympanic

Physical examination:

Diffusely decreased tactile fremitus
Generalized increased resonance on percussion
Distant vesicular breath sounds
Normal capillary refill
No jugular venous distention
No pedal edema
Pulse oximetry 88% with HR 108

ABG physician's office, room air prior to admission:

pH	7.44
$PaCO_2$	32 mmHg
HCO_3	22 mEq/L
PaO_2	52 mmHg
SaO_2	86%

Hematology—CBC:

WBC	9,800/ mm^3
Differential	normal
Hb	15 gm %
Hct	45%

After nasal oxygen: SpO_2 92% with HR 96

Suggested Teaching Points

1. The patient in the video had a thoracoplasty 50 years ago for treatment of tuberculosis. Discuss treatments for tuberculosis in the 1940s and 1950s and how that care can affect patients that RCPs care for today.

2. $\dot{V}/\dot{Q}$ mismatch is one of the causes of hypoxic hypoxia. Discuss the four aspects of $\dot{V}/\dot{Q}$ matching: normal, silent unit, shunt, and dead space.

3. Results of Mr. Feder's CBC are shown. Discuss the significance of a normal WBC and differential in a patient with COPD and new-onset dyspnea and hypoxemia to help rule out an infectious process as the cause of the symptoms. Discuss the importance of assessing hemoglobin and hematocrit values and their relationship to oxygen-carrying capacity.

4. Review application of assessment findings to a therapist-driven protocol for oxygen therapy. If your hospital uses its own TDP, apply these assessment findings to your own protocol.

5. Discuss the pathophysiology of COPD and how it affects oxygenation.

6. Discuss evaluation of patients receiving oxygen therapy: physical assessment, pulse oximetry, ABG, subjective and objective assessment findings.

7. Describe how to use a numerical scale for assessing dyspnea rather than relying on patient responses such as "I feel better" or "I feel worse."

8. Review appropriate patient teaching about oxygen therapy.

9. Discuss setting goals (establishing outcomes) for oxygen therapy. Goals should be measurable, and criteria for assessing progress toward the goal should be included. (Example: improve oxygenation as reflected in pulse oximetry readings)

10. In this case, a nasal cannula was used to administer oxygen. Discuss other alternatives for this patient, such as Venti-mask, etc.

Student Workbook Topics

Oxygenation
Oxygen Delivery
Analysis of Oxygenation
Follow-up to Mr. Feder
Oxygen Therapy Posttest

References

American Association for Respiratory Care: Clinical practice guideline: oxygen therapy in the acute care hospital, Resp Care 36:1410-1413, 1991.

American College of Chest Physicians: National Heart, Lung, and Blood Institute: National conference on oxygen therapy, Resp Care 29:922-935, 1984.

Barnes TA: Core textbook of respiratory care practice, ed 2, St. Louis, 1994, Mosby.

Burton GG, Hodgkin JE, and Ward JJ, editors: Respiratory care: a guide to clinical practice, ed 3, Philadelphia, 1991, JB Lippincott Co.

DesJardins T and Burton GG: Clinical manifestations and assessment of respiratory disease, ed 3, St. Louis, 1995, Mosby.

Dettenmeier PA: Pulmonary nursing care, St. Louis, 1992, Mosby.

Scanlan CL, Spearman CB, and Sheldon RL, editors: Egan's fundamentals of respiratory care, ed 6, St. Louis, 1995, Mosby.

Wilkins RL, Krider SJ, and Sheldon RL, editors: Clinical assessment in respiratory care, ed 3, St. Louis, 1995, Mosby.

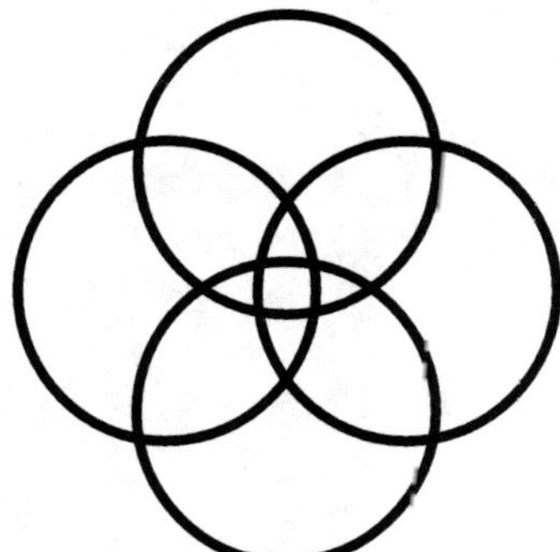

Aerosol Therapy

Learning Objectives

At the end of this program, the learner should be able to...

Knowledge

...recognize the SVN, DPI, MDI devices.
...list three components to the pathophysiology of asthma.
...identify red, yellow, and green zones for PEFR outlined by the National Asthma Education and Prevention Program.

Comprehension

...describe Mr.Carr's breath sounds.
...summarize Mr. Carr's chief complaint, history of present illness, and past medical history.
...explain factors present in Mr. Carr's assessment which reflect his anxiety.

Application

...apply Mr. Carr's assessment findings to a bronchodilator therapy protocol.
...write Mr. Carr's assessment findings according to affiliated hospital policy and procedure for format.
...prepare goals of bronchodilator therapy for Mr. Carr.

Analysis

...compare and contrast Mr. Carr's statements (symptoms, subjective findings) with examination findings (signs, objective findings).
...compare and contrast techniques for use of SVN, MDI, and DPI.
...analyze Mr. Carr's response to therapy.

Synthesis

...formulate a plan of care for Mr. Carr, based on assessment findings.
...develop a teaching plan for Mr. Carr.
...explain why a normal or rising $PaCO_2$ is so serious in a patient with an asthma exacerbation.

Evaluation

...evaluate the results of interventions for Mr. Carr.
...reassess the appropriateness of Mr. Carr's care plan.
...recommend the next step in Mr. Carr's respiratory care.

Video Outline

- I. Introduction
  - A. Historical perspective on aerosol therapy
- II. Assessment
  - A. Referral from nurse
    1. Vital signs
    2. ABG
  - B. RCP interview
    1. Chief complaint
    2. History of present illness
    3. Past medical history
  - C. Physical examination
    1. Pulse oximetry
    2. Inspection
    3. Auscultation
    4. PEFR
  - D. Discussion
    1. Mr. Carr's anxiety
       - a. Appearing fidgety; speaking quickly
       - b. Concerns about multiple issues
       - c. Exaggeration of symptoms
       - d. Daily use of inhaler despite normal PEFR
       - e. RCP response
- III. Analysis
  - A. Asthma
    1. Airway obstruction
       - a. Airway inflammation
         - (1) Anti-inflammatory medications
       - b. Bronchoconstriction
       - c. Mucus secretion
       - d. Decreases in expiratory airflow
       - e. Air trapping
         - (1) Increased FRC
    2. Hypoxemia
       - a. $\dot{V}/\dot{Q}$ mismatch
    3. National Asthma Education and Prevention Program
       - a. Inhaled beta-two agonists
       - b. Systemic corticosteroids
  - B. Aerosol therapy
    1. Aerosol deposition
       - a. Aerosol production and particle characteristics
         - (1) MMAD
         - (2) Nebulizer (SVN)
           - (a) Advantages
           - (b) Disadvantages
         - (3) MDI
           - (a) Advantages
           - (b) Disadvantages
         - (4) DPI
           - (a) Advantages

(b) Disadvantages
b. Patient ventilatory pattern
(1) Recommended patterns
(a) Nebulizer (SVN)
(b) MDI
(c) DPI
c. Airway anatomy and geometry
(1) Deposition patterns

IV. Synthesis
A. MDI/DPI generally preferred
B. General factors leading to consideration of alternate devices
C. Specific factors in Mr. Carr's case resulting in choice of device for beta-two agonist
1. Reduced IC
2. Inability to hold breath
3. Tachypnea
4. Patient request
D. Therapist-driven protocol for bronchodilator
1. Nebulizer (SVN)
E. Goals of therapy
1. Improvement in expiratory airflow
2. Reduction of dyspnea

V. Action
A. Administration of SVN bronchodilator therapy
B. Reassessment
1. PEFR
2. BS

VI. Summary

Video Assessment Findings

Initial nursing assessment:
T 99.2, HR 102, RR 32, BP 130/82

ABG physician's office, room air

pH	7.51
$PaCO_2$	29 mmHg
HCO_3	23
PaO_2	73 mmHg
SaO_2	94%

Physical examination:
Pulse oximetry 96% with HR 105
Solu-Medrol being administered IV
High-pitched, musical inspiratory, and expiratory wheezes throughout both lungs
PEFR approximately 350 L/sec

After treatment:
PEFR approximately 450 L/sec
Wheezes lower-pitched with better aeration

Suggested Teaching Points

1. Since time is limited in video, PEFR was measured only once each time it was assessed. Review proper technique for PEFR measurements.

2. For instructional purposes, the interview and auscultation were detailed and complete. Discuss the clinical decision an RCP might make to shorten the process for a patient in distress.

3. Discuss how sputum production should be evaluated in an asthma patient. Include an expected time frame for sputum production.

4. Discuss the art of assessing wheezing in asthma patients. Include the significance of pitch of wheezes, length of expiratory phase, and significance of localized findings.

5. Ask students to develop guidelines to direct their approach to an anxious patient.

6. Discuss the National Asthma Education and Preventioon Program recommendations for asthma management, with special emphasis on the PRN use of beta-two agonist inhalers. Explore the dilemma RCPs face when they know the current recommendations, yet physicians in their practice area do not follow them.

7. Discuss common misconceptions and myths about asthma (NAEPP pp. 51,59), such as the following: people with asthma should not exercise; asthma is a psychological illness.

8. Discuss evaluation of patients receiving bronchodilator therapy: physical assessment, PEFR, subjective/objective assessment findings.

9. Review appropriate patient teaching about aerosol therapy and use of bronchodilators.

10. Discuss setting goals (establishing outcomes) for aerosol bronchodilator therapy. Goals should be measurable, and criteria for assessing progress toward the goal should be included. (Example: reduce airway obstruction as reflected in PEFR readings)

Student Workbook Topics

Aerosol Therapy Equipment
Bland Aerosol Administration
Follow-up to Mr. Carr
Aerosol Therapy Posttest

References

American Association for Respiratory Care: Aerosol consensus statement, Resp Care 36:916-921, 1991.

American Association for Respiratory Care: Clinical practice guideline: selection of aerosol delivery device, Resp Care 37:891-897, 1992.

Barnes TA: Core textbook of respiratory care practice, ed 2, St. Louis, 1994, Mosby.

DesJardins T and Burton GG: Clinical manifestations and assessment of respiratory disease, ed 3, St. Louis, 1995, Mosby.

Giordano SP: Aerosol therapy: the hard questions, Resp Care 36:914 -915, 1991.

Hess D: Reflections on unanswered questions about aerosol therapy delivery techniques, Resp Care 33:19-20, 1988.

Kacmarek RM and Hess D: The interface between patient and aerosol generator, Resp Care 36:952-973, 1991.

McPherson SP: Respiratory care equipment, ed 5, St. Louis, 1995, Mosby.

National Heart, Lung, and Blood Instittute: Global initiative for asthma, Bethesda, MD, 1995, Publication number 95-3659, National Institutes of Health.

National Heart, Lung, and Blood Institute: Guidelines for the diagnosis and management of asthma, Bethesda, MD, 1991, Publication number 91-3042, National Institutes of Health.

Rau JL: Respiratory care pharmacology, ed 4, St. Louis, 1994, Mosby.

Scanlan CL, Spearman CB, and Sheldon RL, editors: Egan's fundamentals of respiratory care, ed 6, St. Louis, 1995, Mosby.

Wilkins RL, Krider SJ, and Sheldon RL: Clinical assessment in respiratory care, ed 3, St. Louis, 1995, Mosby.

For more information about and literature from the National Asthma Education and Prevention Program, call (301) 251-1222.

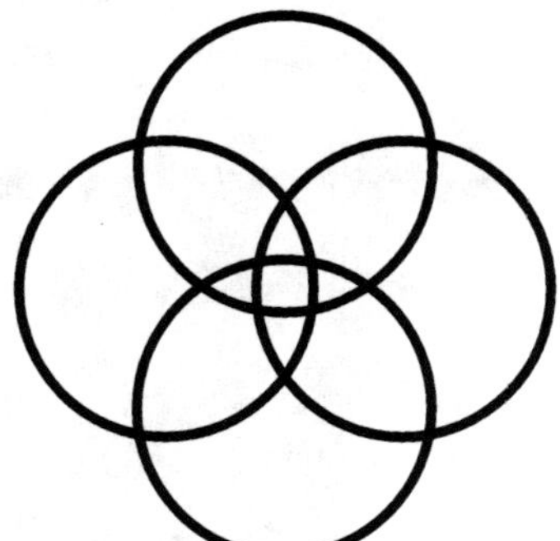

Secretion Management

Learning Objectives

At the end of this program, the learner should be able to...

Knowledge

...recall how pulmonary secretions are normally produced.
...list four factors which impair mucociliary transport.
...name five contraindications to chest physiotherapy.

Comprehension

...describe Mr. Gonsalves' breath sounds.
...summarize Mr. Gonsalves' chief complaint, history of present illness, and past medical history.
...explain factors present in Mr. Gonsalves which impair mucociliary transport.

Application

...apply Mr. Gonsalves' assessment findings to a pulmonary hygiene protocol.
...predict underlying pathophysiology, based on Mr. Gonsalves' assessment findings.
...write goals of pulmonary hygiene therapy for Mr. Gonsalves.

Analysis

...categorize the factors that impair Mr. Gonsalves' mucociliary transport into two categories: (1) those that can be treated or partially reversed during hospital care and (2) those that cannot.
...separate relevant from irrelevant findings in Mr. Gonsalves' history and physical assessment.
...analyze Mr. Gonsalves' response to therapy.

Synthesis

...formulate a plan of care for Mr. Gonsalves, based on assessment findings.
...develop a teaching plan for Mr. Gonsalves.
...prepare all equipment necessary to administer therapy to Mr. Gonsalves.

Evaluation

...evaluate the results of interventions for Mr. Gonsalves.
...reassess the appropriateness of Mr. Gonsalves' care plan.
...recommend the next step in Mr. Gonsalves' respiratory care.

Video Outline

I. Introduction
  A. Impact of reimbursement on care
II. Assessment
  A. Referral from nurse
    1. Vital signs
  B. Chart review
    1. Microbiology
    2. Chest x-ray
    3. ABG
    4. CBC
  C. RCP interview
    1. Chief complaint
    2. History of present illness
    3. Past medical history
  D. Physical examination
    1. Pulse oximetry
    2. Inspection
    3. Palpation
    4. Percussion
    5. Auscultation
      a. Breath sounds
      b. Egophony
  E. Discussion
    1. Chart review relating assessment to pneumonia diagnosis
      a. Microbiology report
      b. CBC
        (1) Leukocytosis
        (2) WBC differential
        (3) Hemoglobin and hematocrit
      c. ABG
      d. CXR
        (1) RML infiltrate
    2. Physical assessment
      a. Tachypnea
      b. Increased fremitus
      c. Dull percussion note
      d. Bronchial/tubular BS
      e. Egophony
III. Analysis
  A. Pneumonia
    1. Host resistance
    2. Virulence
    3. Pathophysiology
      a. Intense tissue reaction
      b. $\dot{V}/\dot{Q}$ mismatch and shunt effect
  B. Pulmonary secretions
    1. Normal condition
    2. Impaired mucociliary transport
      a. Cigarette smoking

b. Dehydration
c. COPD
d. Acute infections
e. Medications

IV. Synthesis
 A. Therapist-driven protocol for pulmonary hygiene
  1. Mr. Gonsalves' findings applied to the protocol
  2. Postural drainage and percussion
 B. Contraindications to therapy
  1. Increased ICP
  2. Head and neck injury or surgery
  3. Uncontrolled airway
  4. Aspiration risk
  5. Abnormal coagulation
  6. Bone disease
 C. Goals of therapy
  1. Increase expectorated sputum to over 30 ml per day
  2. Reduce tubular BS
  3. Reduce crackles
  4. Increase ease of clearing secretions
  5. Decrease infiltrate on CXR

V. Action
 A. Bronchodilator MDI
 B. Segmental breathing
 C. Cough instruction
 D. Postural drainage/percussion
 E. Reassessment after therapy

VI. Summary
 A. Controversy about pulmonary hygiene therapy

Video Assessment Findings

Initial nursing assessment:

T 104.5, HR 108, RR 32 (shallow), BP 160/95

Microbiology:

sputum, good-quality specimen, gram-positive cocci

CXR:

Multiple views demonstrate alveolar infiltrate . . . in the right middle lobe. This appearance is most suggestive of right middle lobe pneumonia. The remainder of the lung fields are clear of alveolar infiltrate.

ABG room air, ED:

pH	7.32
$PaCO_2$	56 mmHg
HCO_3	35 mEq/L
PaO_2	55 mmHg
SaO_2	86%

Hematology—CBC:

WBC	17,500/mm^3
Neutrophil	85
Lymphocyte	10
Monocyte	2
Eosinophil	2
Band	1
Hgb	15.5 gm/dL
Hct	46.5%

Physical examination:

Pulse oximetry 92% with HR 96–100
Penicillin G antibiotic IV
Increased tactile fremitus RML
Dull percussion note RML
Breath sounds:
Posterior: normal vesicular sounds
Anterior: crackles with tubular sounds over RML
Positive egophony

After therapy—breath sounds:

Anterior: crackles no longer present, tubular sounds over RML remaining
Posterior: normal vesicular sounds

Suggested Teaching Points

1. Discuss the difference between relative contraindications and absolute contraindications to therapy and the concept of risk/benefit ratio.
2. Discuss the importance of adequate hydration for all patients with COPD—but particularly for those with pneumonia.
3. Egophony is demonstrated in the physical assessment segment of the video. Discuss the underlying pathophysiology responsible for this finding.
4. Since sputum production is the goal of postural drainage and percussion therapy, discuss using sputum production volume as an assessment tool to determine if therapy is effective.
5. In this case, pulmonary hygiene measures used include segmental breathing, cough instruction, and postural drainage and percussion. Discuss additional therapies such as inhaled Mucomyst (acetylcysteine) and PEP therapy.
6. Review application of assessment findings to a therapist-driven protocol for pulmonary hygiene therapy. If your hospital uses its own TDP, apply these assessment findings to your own protocol.
7. Review appropriate patient teaching about pulmonary hygiene therapy.
8. Discuss setting goals (establishing outcomes) for pulmonary hygiene therapy. Goals should be measurable, and criteria for assessing progress toward the goal should be included. (Example: increase the amount of expectorated sputum to over 30 ml per day, as evidenced by sputum collection in a bedside specimen cup)

9. Discuss safety issues related to administration of chest postural drainage: side rails up, call bell available if RCP leaves room, etc.

10. Discuss use of bronchodilator therapy prior to administration of CPT/PD.

11. Provide a historical perspective on the use of CPT/PD by RCPs. Address controversies that exist today.

Student Workbook Topics

Mucociliary Transport
Pneumonia
Chest Physical Therapy
Follow-up to Mr. Gonsalves
Secretion Management Posttest

References

American Association for Respiratory Care: Clinical practice guideline: postural drainage therapy, Resp Care 36:1418-1426, 1991.

Barnes TA: Core textbook of respiratory care practice, ed 2, St. Louis, 1994, Mosby.

DesJardins T and Burton GG: Clinical manifestations and assessment of respiratory disease, ed 3, St. Louis, 1995, Mosby.

Dettenmeier PA: Pulmonary nursing care, St. Louis, 1992, Mosby.

McCance KL and Huether SE: Pathophysiology: the biologic basis for disease in adults and children, ed 2, St. Louis, 1994, Mosby.

Price SA and Wilson LM: Pathophysiology: clinical concepts of disease processes, ed 4, St. Louis, 1992, Mosby.

Scanlan CL, Spearman CB, and Sheldon RL, editors: Egan's fundamentals of respiratory care, ed 6, St. Louis, 1995, Mosby.

Wilkins RL, Krider SJ, and Sheldon RL, editors: Clinical assessment in respiratory care, ed 3, St. Louis, 1995, Mosby.

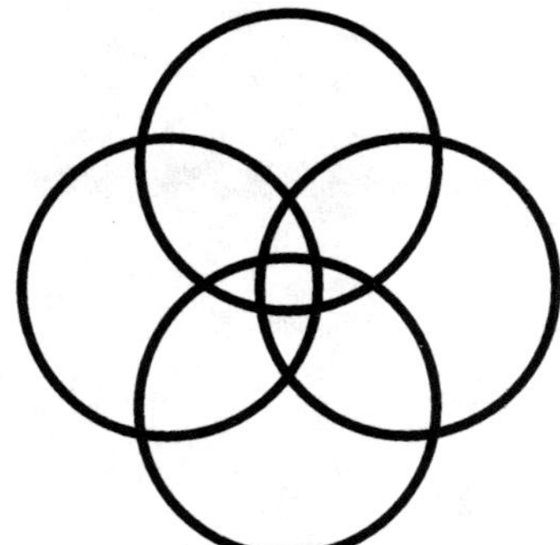

Volume Expansion

Learning Objectives

At the end of this program, the learner should be able to...

Knowledge

...name five changes in the respiratory system associated with aging.
...list four factors that put patients at risk for postoperative respiratory complications.
...state two therapy options to enhance pulmonary volume postoperatively.

Comprehension

...describe Mrs. Howell's breath sounds.
...summarize Mrs. Howell's chief complaint, history of present illness, and past medical history.
...explain how Mrs. Howell's pain can affect her respiratory status.

Application

...apply Mrs. Howell's assessment findings to a therapist-driven protocol for prophylaxis of pulmonary complications.
...write Mrs. Howell's assessment findings according to affiliated hospital policy and procedure for format.
...prepare goals of volume expansion therapy for Mrs. Howell.

Analysis

...categorize the five risk factors for postoperative pulmonary complications into two categories: (1) those that are present in Mrs. Howell and (2) those that are not present.
...separate relevant from irrelevant findings in Mrs. Howell's history and physical examination.
...analyze Mrs Howell's response to therapy.

Synthesis

...formulate a plan of care for Mrs. Howell, based on assessment findings.
...develop a teaching plan for Mrs. Howell.
...explain how Mrs. Howell's attitude will affect her postoperative course.

Evaluation

...evaluate the results of interventions for Mrs. Howell.
...reassess the appropriateness of Mrs. Howell's care plan.
...recommend the next step in Mrs. Howell's respiratory care.

Video Outline

- I. Introduction
  - A. Historical perspective
    - 1. IPPB
    - 2. Incentive spirometry
- II. Assessment
  - A. Referral from nurse
  - B. Chart review
    - 1. PFT
    - 2. ABG
      - a. Preop results
      - b. Postop results
    - 3. Chest x-ray
    - 4. Vital signs
  - C. RCP interview
    - 1. Current condition
    - 2. Past medical history
  - D. Physical examination
    - 1. Inspection
    - 2. Palpation
    - 3. Percussion
    - 4. Auscultation
  - E. Discussion
    - 1. Normal changes with aging
      - a. Decreased elastic recoil
      - b. Fibrotic changes
      - c. Stiffening of chest wall
      - d. Small airway collapse, larger airway dilation (increased V_{DS})
      - e. Enlarged alveoli, decreased in number
      - f. Decreased respiratory muscle strength
      - g. Increased $\dot{V}/\dot{Q}$ mismatch
      - h. 20% drop in PaO_2
      - i. Lower flowrates on PFTs
      - j. Reduced ciliary activity
    - 2. Mental status examination
- III. Analysis
  - A. Atelectasis
    - 1. Airway obstruction
    - 2. Altered sigh
      - a. Alveolar collapse
  - B. Postoperative risk factors
    - 1. Increased secretions
      - a. Smoking
      - b. Intubation
      - c. Inhalation anesthetics
    - 2. Dry, sticky secretions
    - 3. Decreased thoracic expansion
      - a. Postop pain
      - b. Obesity
      - c. Abdominal binders

4. Decreased diaphragmatic mobility
    a. Abdominal distension
    b. Incisional pain
5. Respiratory center depression
    a. Sedatives and narcotics
6. Psychosocial issues

C. Therapy options
1. IPPB
    a. Positive pressure
2. Incentive spirometry
    a. Negative intrathoracic pressure
    b. Patient feedback

D. Matching therapy to patient
1. Incentive spirometry
    a. Indications
    b. Advantages
    c. Requirements
2. IPPB
    a. Indications

IV. Synthesis
A. Risk factors which apply to Mrs. Howell
B. Therapist-driven protocol for a prophylaxis protocol for pulmonary complications
1. Mrs. Howell's findings applied to protocol
C. Goals of therapy
1. Improved breath sounds
2. Absent atelectasis
3. Increased inspiratory capacity

V. Action
A. Administering incentive spirometry
B. Segmental breathing

VI. Summary

Video Assessment Findings

Pulmonary function screening:

	Patient	Predicted	%
FVC	2.69L	2.74L	98%
FEV_1	2.11L		
FEV_1/FVC			82%
$FEF_{25\text{-}75\%}$	1.90 L/s	1.95 L/s	97%

ABG pre-op readings:

pH	7.41
$PaCO_2$	42 mm Hg
HCO_3	28 mEq/L
PaO_2	73 mm Hg
SaO_2	94%

ABG post-op room-air:

pH	7.40
$PaCO_2$	44 mm Hg

HCO_3	27 mEq/L
PaO_2	62 mm Hg
SaO_2	92%

Chest x-ray:

Normal portable film
Central line in proper position

Transfer vital signs:

HR 82, RR 20, BP 122/78, T 99.2 tympanic

Physical examination:

Moderately decreased tactile fremitus
Normal percussion resonance
Normal vesicular breath sounds—initially decreased aeration in bases, increased with encouragement

Suggested Teaching Points

1. In this video, a flow incentive spirometer was used instead of a volume incentive spirometer. Discuss the differences between the two, as well as advantages and disadvantages of each.

2. Perhaps more than any other therapy, patient coaching and teaching is critical to the success of incentive spirometry. Discuss why this is true and what steps the RCP can take to enhance the success of therapy.

3. Discuss why a psychosocial assessment and an assessment of mental status is important when choosing a therapy for postoperative pulmonary volume expansion.

4. Discuss the different methods of postoperative pain control used today: PRN opioids, patient-controlled analgesia, and epidural analgesia. Discuss the effect each is likely to have on the pulmonary system and the risk of postoperative pulmonary complications.

5. Discuss why segmental breathing is a good adjunct to incentive spirometry therapy.

6. Discuss why collaboration with nursing staff is important for the success of incentive spirometry therapy. Ask students to develop strategies to enhance this collaboration.

7. There are still patients for whom IPPB is indicated and appropriate therapy. Ask students to develop their own case studies representing this patient population.

8. Discuss evaluation of patients receiving volume-expansion therapy: physical assessment, IC, subjective/objective assessment findings.

9. Discuss setting goals (establishing outcomes) for volume-expansion therapy. Goals should be measurable, and criteria for assessing progress toward the goal should be included. (Example: enhance deep breathing, as reflected in increasing inspiratory capacity)

Student Workbook Topics

Pathophysiology of Atelectasis
Incentive Spirometry
Intermittent Positive Pressure Breathing
Positive Airway Pressure Breathing
Follow-up to Mrs. Howell
Volume Expansion Posttest

References

American Association for Respiratory Care: Clinical practice guideline: incentive spirometry, Resp Care 36:1402-1405, 1991.

American Association for Respiratory Care: Clinical practice guideline: intermittent positive pressure breathing, Resp Care 38:1189-1195, 1993.

Barnes TA: Core textbook of respiratory care practice, ed 2, St. Louis, 1994, Mosby.

Egan DF: Fundamentals of respiratory therapy, ed 2, St. Louis, 1973, Mosby.

Maas M, Buckwalter KC, and Hardy M: Nursing diagnoses and interventions for the elderly, Redwood City, CA, 1991, Addison-Wesley.

McPherson SP: Respiratory care equipment, ed 5, St. Louis, 1995, Mosby.

Phipps WJ, Long BC, Woods NF, and Cassmeyer VL, editors: Medical-surgical nursing: concepts and clinical practice, ed 4, St. Louis, 1991, Mosby.

Scanlan CL, Spearman CB, and Sheldon RL, editors: Egan's fundamentals of respiratory care, ed 6, St. Louis, 1995, Mosby.

Shapiro BA, Peruzzi WT, and Templin R: Clinical application of blood gases, ed 5, St. Louis, 1994, Mosby.

Wilkins RL, Krider SJ, and Sheldon RL, editors: Clinical assessment in respiratory care, ed 3, St. Louis, 1995, Mosby.

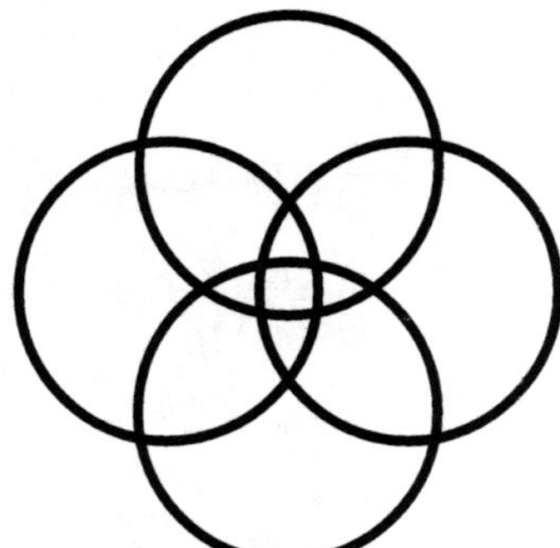

Physical Assessment

Learning Objectives

At the end of this program, the learner should be able to...

Knowledge

...name the three key initial assessments for a trauma patient.
...recall the first intervention provided by the RCP for this patient.
...state two complaints this patient had about his respiratory condition.

Comprehension

...describe Mr. Donovan's breath sounds.
...summarize Mr. Donovan's chief complaint, history of present illness, and past medical history.
...explain how Mr. Donovan's accident could have caused chest injuries.

Application

...apply Mr. Donovan's assessment findings to a therapist-driven trauma protocol.
...write Mr. Donovan's assessment findings according to affiliated hospital policy and procedure for format.
...illustrate the difference between an open and closed pneumothorax.

Analysis

...compare and contrast the physical findings and potential complications of open and closed pneumothorax.
...separate primary from secondary assessments of the trauma patient.
...analyze Mr. Donovan's response to initial trauma interventions.

Synthesis

...formulate a plan of care for Mr. Donovan, based on assessment findings.
...develop a teaching plan for Mr. Donovan.
...explain the concept of mechanism of injury—and the mechanism of injury responsible for Mr. Donovan's injuries.

Evaluation

...evaluate the results of interventions for Mr. Donovan.
...reassess the appropriateness of Mr. Donovan's care plan.
...recommend the next step in Mr. Donovan's respiratory care.

Video Outline

I. Introduction
II. Assessment
  A. Nurse's report to RCP
  B. Physical examination
    1. Pulse oximetry
    2. Inspection
    3. Palpation
    4. Percussion
    5. Auscultation
      a. Lungs
      b. Heart
  C. Past medical history
  D. Summary by RCP to nurse
  E. Discussion
    1. Primary assessment
      a. Airway
        (1) Risk factors for airway obstruction
          (a) C-spine immobilization
          (b) Intoxication
          (c) Vomiting
          (d) Head injuries
          (e) Decreased LOC
          (f) Soft-tissue swelling
      b. Breathing
        (1) Observation/inspection
      c. Circulation
        (1) Capillary refill
        (2) BP
        (3) Tissue oxygenation
    2. Secondary assessment
      a. Inspection
        (1) Face
        (2) Neck
          (a) Risk/benefit of removing c-collar
      b. Palpation
        (1) Skin temperature and moisture
        (2) Stability of bony thoracic cage
        (3) Pain
      c. Percussion
        (1) Hyper- or hyporesonance
      d. Auscultation
        (1) Lung
        (2) Heart
III. Analysis
  A. Mechanism of injury
    1. Deceleration forces
      a. Types of deceleration injuries
      b. Injury at hilum and pleura
  B. Pneumothorax

1. Definition
2. Normal anatomy and physiology
3. Open
4. Closed
5. Tension pneumothorax

C. Application to Mr. Donovan
D. Oxygen-carrying capacity
   1. Circulation

IV. Synthesis
   A. Oxygen administration
   B. Review of Mr. Donovan's care while following trauma protocol
      1. Airway
      2. Breathing
      3. Oxygen administration
   C. Goals of therapy

V. Action
   A. Reassessment
      1. EKG/pulse ox monitor
      2. CXR
         a. Pneumothorax
         b. S/P chest tube with lung reexpanded
      3. Chest drain
      4. Switch to nasal cannula

VI. Summary

Video Assessment Findings

Initial nursing assessment:
HR 124, BP 90/62
Positive blood-alcohol level
No loss of consciousness

Pulse oximetry on room air: 88% with HR 128

Physical examination:
Left side of chest not moving as much as right side on inspection
Capillary refill normal
No cyanosis
Percussion of anterior lung fields: lightly increased resonance over left upper chest
Breath sounds: normal vesicular—slightly diminished aeration, left upper anterior chest
Heart tones normal

Pulse oximetry with oxygen: 95% with HR 105

ABG after chest tube:

pH	7.41
$PaCO_2$	34 mm Hg
HCO_3	21 mEq/L
PaO_2	317 mm Hg
SaO_2	99%

Monitor display:

HR	sinus rhythm at 85/min
RR	26
SpO_2	98%
BP	122/93

Chest x-rays:

first x-ray: 25% tension pneumothorax on left, noted with markings on film
Note: D-shaped artifact over heart is the ring for the strap on the sling.
second x-ray (after chest tube): resolution of pneumothorax, lung reexpanded

Chest drain bubbling in water-seal chamber with cough only

Suggested Teaching Points

1. Mr. Donovan's blood pressure increased from 90/62 to 122/93 during this case presentation. Discuss fluid resuscitation in trauma patients and how administering fluids and treating a pneumothorax with chest drainage can improve blood pressure.

2. Collaborate with a trauma nurse or physician to teach students about the overall care of the trauma patient and how respiratory care is integrated into that care. Also discuss the concept of mechanism of injury.

3. Discuss the concept of primary and secondary assessments and interventions in trauma patients. The trauma protocol in the workbook appendix outlines primary assessments and interventions; have students develop a protocol for secondary respiratory assessments and interventions. You may again wish to collaborate with an emergency care professional.

4. Discuss how poor perfusion (hypotension or shock) will affect pulse oximetry readings. Include topics such as correlation between apical heart rate and heart rate displayed on the monitor, pulse strength indicator on monitor, and correlation with ABG.

5. Since it is very difficult to show detail of chest x-rays on video, collect actual films from patients with pneumothorax. Review them with special emphasis on identifying the lung border, the lack of lung markings in the periphery of the affected side, and the differences in densities between the affected and unaffected side.

6. Provide a more detailed discussion of chest drainage to supplement the brief inspection in the video. Additional resources from the literature are included in this case's bibliography.

7. Discuss the relationship between blood loss in trauma and oxygen-carrying capacity. Point out how tissue hypoxia can occur from lack of circulation, even when the PaO_2 is high.

8. In the video, the patient had significant pain on palpation of the left upper chest, and during inspection of the chest, the right side moved more than the left during breathing. Discuss the concept of splinting due to pain, as well as the impact splinting can have on pulmonary function.

Student Workbook Topics

Initial Patient Assessment
Vital Signs
Chest Physical Assessment
Chest Trauma
Chest Drainage
Assessment of the Trauma Patient
Follow-up to Mr. Donovan
Physical Assessment/Chest Trauma Posttest

References

Carroll P: Chest tubes made easy, RN 58:46-56, 1995.

Carroll PF: Chest tubes and pleural drainage, AARC Individual Independent Study Package, Dallas, 1992, AARC.

Gordon PA, Norton JM, and Merrell R: Refining chest tube management: analysis of the state of practice, DCCN 14:6-12, 1995.

Gross SB: Current challenges, concepts, and controversies in chest tube management, AACN Clin Issues Crit Care Nurs 4:260-275, 1993.

Rea R, editor: Trauma nursing core course (provider) manual, ed 3, Chicago, 1991, Emergency Nurses Association.

Sheehy SB: Emergency nursing principles and practice, ed 3, St. Louis, 1992, Mosby.

Sheehy SB: Manual of emergency care, ed 3, St. Louis, 1990, Mosby.

Taliaferro E: Disease and trauma monographs for acute care: pneumothorax, Emergindex®, vol 86, Denver, 1995, Micromedix, Inc.

Wilkins RL, Krider SJ, and Sheldon RL, editors: Clinical assessment in respiratory care, ed 3, St. Louis, 1995, Mosby.

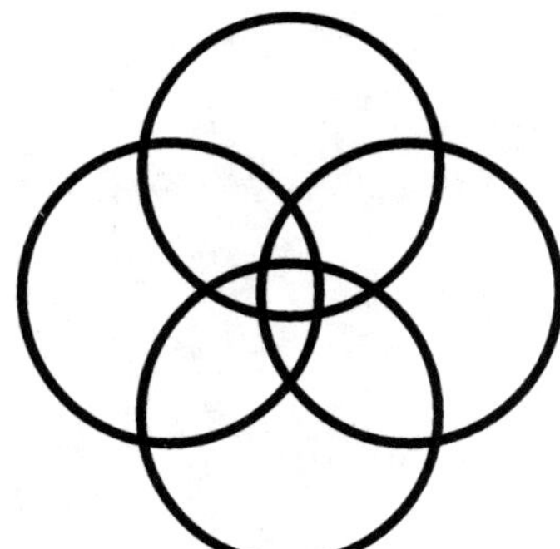

Pediatrics

Learning Objectives

At the end of this program, the learner should be able to...

Knowledge

...identify proper positioning to open an infant's airway.
...define croup and epiglottitis.
...label the following structures on a diagram of the upper airway: tongue, epiglottis, larynx, vocal cords, subglottic area, trachea.

Comprehension

...describe the sounds heard on auscultation of Alyssa's neck.
...summarize Alyssa's chief complaint, history of present illness, and past medical history.
...contrast the signs and symptoms seen with croup to those seen with epiglottitis.

Application

...demonstrate an age-appropriate approach to providing respiratory care to Alyssa.
...write Alyssa's assessment findings according to affiliated hospital policy and procedure for format.
...illustrate the difference between the effect of edema in a child's airway compared with an adult's.

Analysis

...compare and contrast the physical findings and pathophysiology of croup and epiglottitis.
...distinguish between appropriate approaches to care of children of various ages.
...diagram the location of the infection in epiglottitis and croup.

Synthesis

...formulate a plan of care for Alyssa, based on her age and assessment findings.
...develop a teaching plan for Alyssa and her mother.
...explain why adequate hydration is so critical in children with respiratory illness.

Evaluation

...evaluate the results of interventions for Alyssa.
...reassess the appropriateness of Alyssa's care plan.
...recommend the next step in Alyssa's respiratory care.

Video Outline

I. Introduction
  A. Age-appropriate care
II. Assessment
  A. RCP interview
    1. History of present illness
    2. Chief complaint
    3. History of present illness—additional information
    4. Past medical history
  B. Physical examination
    1. Pulse oximetry
    2. Auscultation
  C. Chart review
    1. Vital signs
    2. Physician orders
  D. Discussion
    1. Observation of sick child
      a. Behavioral clues
    2. Airway
      a. Child versus adult
        (1) Diameter
        (2) Head and neck
        (3) Tongue
        (4) Positioning
          (a) By RCP
          (b) By child
    3. Breathing
      a. Less pulmonary reserve
    4. Circulation
      a. Compensatory mechanisms
      b. Less cardiac reserve
      c. Intravascular volume critical
    5. Review of this case
      a. Allowing child to remain with caregiver
      b. Not ignoring child
      c. Getting history from adult
      d. Inspection during history
      e. Making judgments about how much action to take with fussy child
      f. Assessment
        (1) Airway
        (2) Breathing
        (3) Circulation
III. Analysis
  A. Epiglottitis
    1. Bacterial infection
      a. *Haemophilus influenzae*
    2. Onset
    3. History
    4. Signs and symptoms
    5. Management

B. Croup
 1. Viral infection
 2. Signs and symptoms
  a. Based on age and airway size
   (1) How edema affects different-sized airways
    (a) Poiseuille's law

IV. Synthesis
 A. Treatment of croup
  1. Systemic steroids
  2. Racemic epinephrine
   a. Rebound
   b. Hospital protocols for discharge after racemic epinephrine
  3. Age-appropriate care
   a. Preschool developmental age
    (1) Characteristics
   b. Approach to Alyssa
    (1) Play—with simulated treatment
  4. Goals of therapy
   a. Reducing airway obstruction

V. Action
 A. Playing with child
 B. Administering aerosol
 C. Reassessment

VI. Summary

Video Assessment Findings

Physical examination:
Pulse oximetry on room air: 96% with HR 120
Inspiratory stridor on auscultation of neck

Admission vital signs:
T 100.2 tympanic, BP 90/60, HR 120, RR 32

Physician order sheet:
Racemic epinephrine via neb
0.5 ml of 2.25% solution now
Prednisolone oral solution
5 mg/ml
Give 6 mg/6 ml PO now

After treatment:
stridor absent

Suggested Teaching Points

1. The video discusses different approaches to providing respiratory care to children, based on their developmental ages. Direct students to additional references such as psychology or pediatric nursing texts to make a chart outlining the developmental ages and key aspects of each. Then, have students write a guide listing approaches to respiratory care for children of various developmental ages.

2. Have RCP students use role-playing to practice caring for children of different ages.

3. Health care professionals must often be creative when dealing with children. Discuss creative alternatives to situations such as these:
   a. A child is frightened of the mask for aerosol therapy and is too young to use a mouthpiece. (Potential solution: use a familar paper cup—it's best if the cup has decorations—and cut a hole in the bottom of the cup, inserting the aerosol tubing into the cup. Then, hold the less-frightening paper cup to the child's face. Tip: put stickers that the child likes in the bottom of the cup to make it more interesting to look at.)
   b. A child has a sore throat and doesn't want to drink. He has a fever and high respiratory rate and is at risk for dehydration. An IV is being considered. What could be offered instead? (Potential solution: give the child a popsicle—the cold will be soothing to his sore throat, and the popsicle is often a special treat to a child. The liquid equivalent will provide hydration.)

4. Discuss the significance of the difference between the finding of inspiratory stridor alone versus inspiratory/expiratory stridor in a child with an upper airway infection.

5. The *Haemophilus infleunzae* vaccine has reduced the number of cases of epiglottitis. Discuss the subject of childhood immunizations and the impact these vaccines have had on childhood respiratory illness (particularly pertussis).

6. Causes of cardiopulmonary arrest in children are different from adults. Discuss how resuscitation of children is different. (Consult American Heart Association's PALS vs. ACLS)

7. This video focused on upper airway infection and obstruction. Discuss how the principles of pediatric care discussed in this video apply to children with illnesses such as asthma, pneumonia, and cystic fibrosis.

Student Workbook Topics

Croup and Epiglottitis
Physiological/Anatomical Pediatric Variations and Care of the Pediatric Patient
Aerosol Delivery in Pediatrics
Follow-up to Alyssa
Pediatrics Posttest

References

Alfaro-LeFevere R, Blicharz ME, Flynn NM, and Boyer MJ: Drug handbook: A nursing process approach, Redwood City, CA, 1992, Addison Wesley.

American Association for Respiratory Care: Clinical practice guideline: delivery of aerosols to the upper airway, Resp Care 39:803-807, 1994.

American Association for Respiratory Care: Clinical practice guideline: selection of an aerosol delivery device for neonatal and pediatric patients, Resp Care 40:1325-1335, 1995.

Barkin RM: Pediatric respiratory emergencies, Emerg Care Q 5:71-78, 1989.

Dershewitz RA, editor: Ambulatory pediatric care, ed 2, Philadelphia, 1993, JB Lippincott.

Haley K and Baker P, editors: Emergency nursing pediatric course instructor manual, Chicago, 1993, Emergency Nurses Association.

Hathaway WE and Groothuis JR, editors: Current pediatric diagnosis and treatment, ed 10, Norwalk, CT, 1991, Appleton and Lange.

Nursing 95: Drug handbook, Springhouse, PA, 1995 Springhouse Corporation.

Rau JL: Delivery of aerosolized drugs to neonatal and pediatric patients, Resp Care 36:514-545, 1991.

Rau JL: Respiratory care pharmacology, ed 4, St. Louis, 1994, Mosby.

Scanlan CL, Spearman CB, and Sheldon RL, editors: Egan's fundamentals of respiratory care, ed 6, St. Louis, 1995, Mosby.

Sly RM: Aerosol therapy in children, Resp Care 36, 994-1007, 1991.

Smith J: Big differences in little people, Am J Nurs 88: 459-462, 1988.

Wong DL: Whaley and Wong's nursing care of infants and children, ed 5, St. Louis, 1994, Mosby.

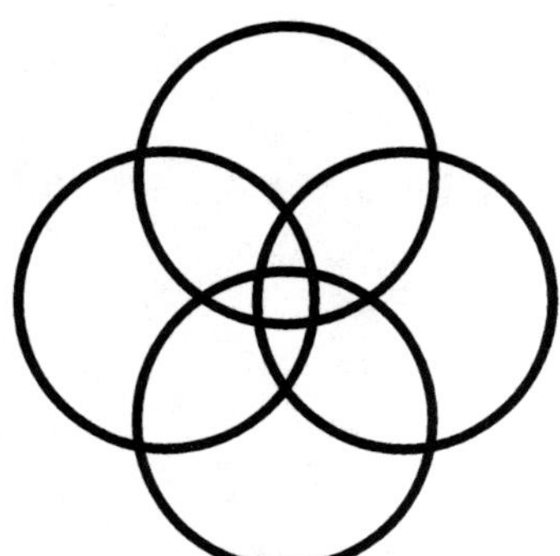

Noninvasive Monitoring

Learning Objectives

At the end of this program, the learner should be able to...

Knowledge

...identify the P, Q, R, S, and T waves on an EKG tracing.
...name six factors that can affect the performance of pulse oximetry monitoring.
...reproduce a normal capnography tracing.

Comprehension

...describe Ms. Reilly's breath sounds.
...summarize Ms. Reilly's chief complaint, history of present illness, and past medical history.
...explain why Ms. Reilly was intubated in the emergency department.

Application

...predict noninvasive monitoring findings that would be associated with a deterioration in Ms. Reilly's condition.
...write Ms. Reilly's assessment findings according to affiliated hospital policy and procedure for format.
...choose noninvasive monitoring devices that would be appropriate to monitor Ms. Reilly's condition.

Analysis

...compare and contrast the data available from pulse oximetry, capnography, and EKG monitoring.
...separate actual data from artifact for the above named monitoring devices.
...analyze Ms. Reilly's noninvasive monitoring findings.

Synthesis

...formulate a plan of care for Ms. Reilly, based on assessment findings.
...develop a teaching plan for Ms. Reilly, her family, and her nurse.
...explain why capnography, EKG, and pulse oximetry monitoring are important for Ms. Reilly.

Evaluation

...evaluate the results of monitoring Ms. Reilly.
...reassess the appropriateness of Ms. Reilly's care plan.
...recommend the next step in Ms. Reilly's respiratory care.

Video Outline

I. Introduction
  A. Historical perspective
II. Assessment
  A. Interview with nurse
    1. History of present illness
      a. Caring for tricyclic overdose patient
      b. ABG
  B. Physical assessment
    1. Tachycardia
    2. Auscultation
    3. Inspection
  C. Discussion with nurse
    1. Past medical history
  D. Discussion
    1. Talking with nurse away from patient bedside
    2. Speak with unconscious patient
    3. Auscultation
      a. Assess ET tube position
    4. Inspection
      a. Position of ET tube
      b. Check oxygen equipment
      c. Look for mist at T-tube
      d. Monitor
III. Analysis
  A. Overdose
    1. Airway
    2. Remove toxic substance
      a. Gastric lavage
      b. Activated charcoal
      c. Magnesium citrate
  B. EKG monitoring
    1. Tracing
      a. P wave
        (1) Location on tracing
        (2) Correlation to physiology
      b. QRS complex
        (1) Location on tracing
        (2) Correlation to physiology
      c. T wave
        (1) Location on tracing
        (2) Correlation to physiology
    2. Application to Ms. Reilly
  C. Capnography
    1. Definition
    2. Tracing
      a. Zero baseline
      b. Rapid, sharp uprise
      c. Alveolar plateau
      d. Well-defined end point

e. Rapid, sharp downstroke
3. Clinical uses
a. Detect esophageal intubation
b. Detect leaks around ET tube cuff
c. Monitor weaning
d. Monitor return of diaphragmatic function after neuromuscular drugs
e. Detect pulmonary embolic events
f. Monitor patients at risk for respiratory depression
D. Pulse oximetry
1. Operating principles
2. Factors affecting performance
a. Motion artifact
b. Abnormal hemoglobin
c. Intravascular dyes
d. Ambient light on sensor
e. Low perfusion
f. Skin pigmentation
g. Nail coverings with finger probe
h. Saturation below 83%
3. Factors affecting interpretation
a. Oxyhemoglobin dissociation curve
b. Compare with ABG
IV. Synthesis
A. Goals of noninvasive monitoring
1. Detect changes early
B. Monitor devices
1. EKG
2. Pulse oximetry
a. Apply factors affecting performance to Ms. Reilly
3. Capnography
a. Factors resulting in misleading trends
(1) Variations in temperature
(2) Variations in cardiovascular function
(3) Variations in carbon dioxide waveform
V. Action
A. Apply pulse oximeter
1. Chooses finger on arm without NIBP
B. Apply capnography sensor
1. Interpretation of waveform
2. Explain interpretation to nurse
VI. Reassessment
A. Therapist-driven protocol for pulse oximetry
1. Ms. Reilly's findings applied to the protocol
B. Discussion with nurse
1. Review of past 24 hours
C. Evaluate for discontinuance of pulse oximetry
1. Apply clinical findings to protocol
VII. Summary

Video Assessment Findings

Monitor display:

EKG sinus tachycardia at 140
BP 112/91

ABGs:

pH 7.37
$PaCO_2$ 41 mm Hg
HCO_3 23 mEq/L
PaO_2 158 mm Hg
SaO_2 99%

Physical examination:

Normal vesicular breath sounds
ET tube: 23 cm mark at lip corner
Oxygen flowmeter at 12 LPM
Oxygen setting on nebulizer: 40%
Mist visible at end of tubing on T-tube
Cardiac monitor as above

Monitor—after application of pulse oximetry:

EKG sinus tachycardia at 140
SaO_2 98
BP 110/91
$EtCO_2$ 39 with RR 14

Note regarding $EtCO_2$ monitor display: the two numbers which appear above the tracing represent minimum CO_2 and respiratory rate. The minimum CO_2 should be zero—to indicate there is a proper zero baseline. The digital display to the right of the tracing indicates actual $EtCO_2$ reading in mm Hg.

Suggested Teaching Points

1. In the video, when the RCP was placing the pulse oximeter sensor on Ms. Reilly's finger, he was initially going to place it on the arm with the noninvasive blood pressure cuff, then placed it on the other arm. Discuss why he did this—why he avoided the arm with the NIBP cuff.

2. Many hospitals today have eliminated the routine use of heaters with large-volume nebulizers. Discuss the pros and cons of this approach.

3. Discuss why the RCP looks for mist at peak inspiration coming out of the distal end of the aerosol tubing attached to the T-piece. Discuss what should be done if the mist disappears.

4. In this video, the end-tidal CO_2 was monitored on an intubated patient. Discuss how this monitoring is accomplished in a nonintubated patient.

5. Provide case studies to match the $EtCO_2$ waveforms and EKG tracings illustrated in the student workbook.

6. Collaborate with an emergency medicine professional to discuss the overall management of overdose patients, with a focus on selected medications commonly seen when patients take a drug overdose. Review different approaches to different medications and implications for the RCP.

7. Discuss assessment of proper ET tube cuff inflation in a patient not receiving mechanical ventilation.

8. In the video, the RCP and nurse discussed the patient's condition away from the bedside, out of earshot of the patient. Use this illustration to reinforce the confidential information RCPs are privy to—and the critical importance of not discussing patients where other patients, families, visitors, and others can hear.

Student Workbook Topics

Electrocardiography
Pulse Oximetry
Capnography
Follow-up to Ms. Reilly
Noninvasive Monitoring Posttest

References

American Association for Respiratory Care: Clinical practice guideline: bland aerosol administration, Resp Care 38:1196-1200, 1993.

American Association for Respiratory Care: Clinical practice guideline: capnography/capnometry during mechanical ventilation, Resp Care 40: 1321-1324, 1995.

American Association for Respiratory Care: Clinical practice guideline: pulse oximetry, Resp Care 36:1406-1409, 1991.

Keough V and McNamara P: Case review: a 27-year-old with a tricyclic overdose, J Emerg Nurs 19: 382-384, 1993.

Krueger K: More on management of patient with tricyclic overdose [letter to the editor], J Emerg Nurs 20: 173-174, 1994.

McPherson SP: Respiratory care equipment, ed 5, St. Louis, 1995, Mosby.

Meltzer LE, Pinneo R, and Kitchell JR: Intensive coronary care: a manual for nurses, Bowie, MD, 1970, The Charles Press.

Nellcor Incorporated: Advanced concepts in capnography, Hayward, CA, 1988, Author.

Nursing 96: Drug handbook, Springhouse, PA, 1996, Springhouse Corporation.

Pilbeam SP: Mechanical ventilation: physiological and clinical applications, ed 2, St. Louis, 1992, Mosby.

Poisindex® editorial staff: Toxicologic management: antidepressants, tricyclic, Poisindex®, vol 86, Denver, 1995, Micromedix, Inc.

Scanlan CL, Spearman CB, and Sheldon RL, editors: Egan's fundamentals of respiratory care, ed 6, St. Louis, 1995, Mosby.

Schmitz BD and Shapiro BA: Capnography, Respiratory Care Clinics of North America 1: 107-117, 1995.

Sheehy SB: Emergency nursing principles and practice, ed 3, St. Louis, 1992, Mosby.
Sheehy SB: Manual of emergency care, ed 3, St. Louis, 1990, Mosby.

Wilkins RL, Krider SJ, and Sheldon RL, editors: Clinical assessment in respiratory care, ed 3, St. Louis, 1995, Mosby.

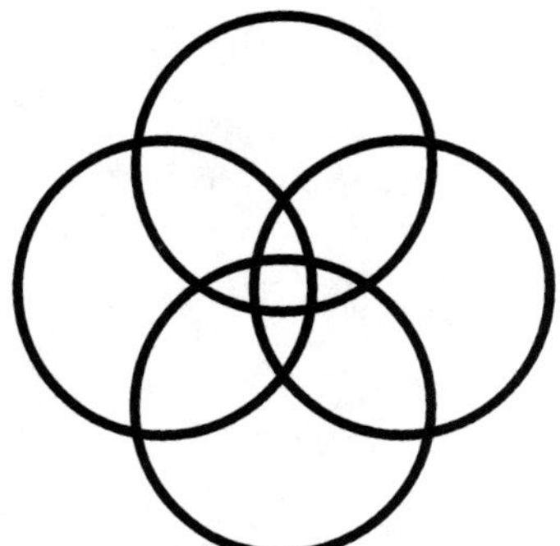

Mechanical Ventilation

Learning Objectives

At the end of this program, the learner should be able to...

Knowledge

...name clinical signs associated with congestive heart failure.
...list four potential benefits of PEEP therapy.
...state two approaches to treatment of cardiogenic pulmonary edema.

Comprehension

...describe Mrs. Gleason's breath sounds.
...summarize Mrs. Gleason's chief complaint, history of present illness, and past medical history.
...explain how Mrs. Gleason's vital signs reflect pathophysiologic changes seen in congestive heart failure.

Application

...apply Mrs. Gleason's assessment findings to a therapist-driven protocol for mechanical ventilation.
...write Mrs. Gleason's assessment findings according to affiliated hospital policy and procedure for format.
...prepare goals of mechanical ventilation therapy for Mrs. Gleason.

Analysis

...categorize the treatments for cardiogenic pulmonary edema into those addressing myocardial performance and those addressing lung fluid.
...diagram the effects of PEEP in the lung.
...analyze Mrs Gleason's response to therapy.

Synthesis

...formulate a plan of care for Mrs. Gleason, based on assessment findings and underlying pathophysiology.
...develop a teaching plan for Mrs. Gleason, her family, and her nurse.
...explain how Mrs. Gleason's myocardial infarction resulted in the changes in her respiratory status.

Evaluation

...evaluate the results of interventions for Mrs. Gleason.
...reassess the appropriateness of Mrs. Gleason's care plan.
...recommend the next step in Mrs. Gleason's respiratory care.

Video Outline

I. Introduction
   A. Historical perspective
II. Assessment
   A. Shift change report
      1. History of present illness
      2. Chief complaint
      3. Past medical history
   B. RCP introduction to patient
   C. Auscultation
      1. Breath sounds
      2. Heart sounds
   D. Inspection of patient
   E. Ventilator check
      1. Mode: SIMV
      2. Tidal volume: 750 ml
      3. Rate: 10
      4. FIO_2: .40
      5. PEEP: 3 cm H_2O
      6. High-pressure limit: 45 cm H_2O
      7. Low tidal volume alarm: 600 ml
      8. Low exhaled volume alarm: 6.0 L
      9. Measured VT
      10. Measured respiratory rate
      11. Measured peak pressure
      12. Peak flow: 40 LPM
      13. Measured compliance
      14. Analyzed FIO_2
      15. Temperature: 37°C
      16. Measured PEEP: 3 cm H_2O
   F. Monitor
      1. SpO_2 decreased
      2. HR increased
   G. Discussion with nurse
      1. Urine output decreased
      2. RCP discussed findings
   H. Auscultation of back
   I. Discussion
      1. Acute respiratory failure
      2. Assess patient first
         a. New crackles
      3. Assess ventilator
         a. Static compliance
            (1) Peak and plateau pressures increased
4. Assess monitor
         a. HR increased
         b. SpO_2 decreased
      5. Assess urine output
      6. Assess posterior breath sounds

- III. Analysis
  - A. Myocardial infarction
    - 1. Pathophysiology
    - 2. Impaired left ventricle function
    - 3. Effects of MI
      - a. Abnormal ventricular wall function
      - b. Altered ventricular compliance
      - c. Reduced stroke volume
    - 4. Factors determining functional impairment
      - a. Size of infarct
      - b. Infarct location
      - c. Condition of myocardium
  - B. Congestive heart failure
    - 1. Pathophysiology
      - a. Starling's law of the heart
      - b. Decreased stroke volume
      - c. Increased heart rate
      - d. Vasoconstriction
    - 2. Clinical signs
      - a. Increased HR
      - b. Normal BP
      - c. Decreased urine output
  - C. Pulmonary edema
    - 1. Pathophysiology
      - a. Offsetting pressures
        - (1) Hydrostatic
        - (2) Oncotic
      - b. Heart failure
      - c. Pulmonary effects
    - 2. Treatment
      - a. Increase myocardial performance
        - (1) Increase contractility
        - (2) Reduce vascular resistance
          - (a) Vasodilators
          - (b) Diuretics
      - b. Reduce fluid in lungs
        - (1) PEEP
          - (a) Increase alveolar volume
          - (b) Redistribute lung water
          - (c) Reopen collapsed or obstructed respiratory bronchioles
          - (d) Improve $\dot{V}/\dot{Q}$ matching
          - (e) Reduce shunting
          - (f) Increase lung compliance
          - (g) Increase lung volumes
- IV. Synthesis
  - A. Apply analysis data to Mrs. Gleason
  - B. Goals of therapy
    - 1. Improve myocardial contractility and cardiac output
    - 2. Specific to mechanical ventilation
      - a. Improve oxygenation
      - b. Maintain adequate ventilation

- C. Therapist-driven protocol for mechanical ventilation
  - 1. Ventilation adequate
  - 2. Protocol says increase FIO_2
    - a. Apply pathophysiology
  - 3. Increase PEEP instead

V. Action

- A. Increase PEEP
- B. Nursing actions
  - 1. Nitroglycerin drip
  - 2. Digitalis
  - 3. Furosemide
- C. Later reassessment
  - 1. Increased urine output
  - 2. Decreased peak pressures
  - 3. Breath sounds
  - 4. Decreased HR
  - 5. Improved compliance

VI. Summary

- A. Apply knowledge of pathophysiology to TDP
- B. Collaborative practice

Video Assessment Findings

Shift change report—ABG on SIMV: 10, VT: 750ml, FIO_2: .40, PEEP: 3 cm H_2O

pH	7.43
$PaCO_2$	37 mm Hg
HCO_3	25 mEq/L
PaO_2	98 mm Hg
SaO_2	97%

Physical examination:

Breath sounds: normal vesicular sounds upper anterior, crackles in dependent areas
Heart sounds: gallop rhythm
ET tube: 23 cm mark at mouth corner

Ventilator flow sheet:

See video outline

Monitor:

EKG	sinus rhythm at 99
SpO_2	92%
BP	122/70

Physical examination:

Breath sounds: crackles throughout posterior lung fields

ABG with clinical changes:

pH	7.41
$PaCO_2$	42 mm Hg
HCO_3	27 mEq/L
PaO_2	70 mm Hg

SaO_2 93%

Physical examination:

Breath sounds: crackles at bases; otherwise, normal vesicular sounds

Monitor:

EKG normal sinus rhythm at 79
SpO_2 97%
BP 133/72

Suggested Teaching Points

1. The assessment segment of this video shows a routine ventilator check. A ventilator flow sheet is in the student workbook. Tell the students to fill out the flow sheet as they watch the video. Or, use the ventilator flow sheet from your clinical affiliate(s).

2. Discuss whether a pulmonary artery catheter is indicated in this patient. Consider the additional information that would be provided. Predict Mrs. Gleason's hemodynamic values. Analyze how that information would be used in a respiratory care plan.

3. The video discusses how a dysfunction in another organ system (cardiovascular) affects the lungs. Discuss how neurological dysfunction can affect the respiratory system.

4. Discuss the difference in pathophysiology between cardiogenic and noncardiogenic pulmonary edema.

5. Discuss the effects of PEEP on the cardiovascular system. Address how PEEP's effects are different in patients with hypotension and/or hypovolemia.

6. Reinforce the concept that TDPs can be used safely and successfully only when the RCP understands the underlying pathophysiology.

7. Collaborate with another critical care professional—physician, registered nurse, or pharmacist—to discuss medications used to treat myocardial infarction and heart failure.

8. Discuss evaluation of patients receiving mechanical ventilation: physical assessment, ABG, compliance, noninvasive monitoring, subjective/objective assessment findings, etc.

9. Discuss setting goals (establishing outcomes) for mechanical ventilation therapy. Goals should be measurable, and criteria for assessing progress toward the goal should be included. (Example: maintain acceptable ventilation, as reflected in arterial pH and $PaCO_2$ values. Discuss the difference between "acceptable" levels and "normal" levels and how patients with COPD may never have "normal" levels.)

Student Workbook Topics

Mechanical Ventilation
PEEP Therapy
Pulmonary Edema, Myocardial Infarction, and Congestive Heart Failure
Follow-up to Mrs. Gleason
Mechanical Ventilation Posttest

References

American Association for Respiratory Care: Clinical practice guideline: patient-ventilator system checks, Resp Care 37: 882-886, 1992.

DesJardins T and Burton GG: Clinical manifestations and assessment of respiratory disease, ed 3, St. Louis, 1995, Mosby.

Keen JH, Baird MS, and Allen JH: Mosby's critical care and emergency drug reference, St. Louis, 1994, Mosby.

McCance KL and Huether SE: Pathophysiology: the biologic basis for disease in adults and children, ed 2, St. Louis, 1994, Mosby.

McPherson SP: Respiratory care equipment, ed 5, St. Louis, 1995, Mosby.

Nursing 95: Drug handbook, Springhouse, PA, 1995 Springhouse Corporation.

Pilbeam SP: Mechanical ventilation: physiological and clinical applications, ed 2, St. Louis, 1992, Mosby.

Price SA and Wilson LM: Pathophysiology: clinical concepts of disease processes, ed 4, St. Louis, 1992, Mosby.

Scanlan CL, Spearman CB, and Sheldon RL, editors: Egan's fundamentals of respiratory care, ed 6, St. Louis, 1995, Mosby.

Society of Critical Care Medicine Task Force on Guidelines: Guidelines for standards of care for patients with acute respiratory failure on mechanical ventilatory support, Crit Care Med 19: 275-278, 1991.

Urban NA, Greenlee KK, Krumberger JM, and Winkelman C: Guidelines for critical care nursing, St. Louis, 1995, Mosby.

Wilkins RL, Krider SJ, and Sheldon RL, editors: Clinical assessment in respiratory care, ed 3, St. Louis, 1995, Mosby.

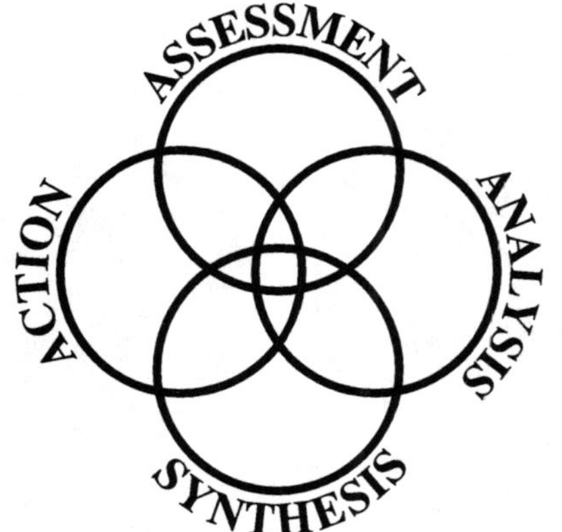

Part II

The Competency Evaluation Series

Competency Evaluation Questions and Suggested Responses

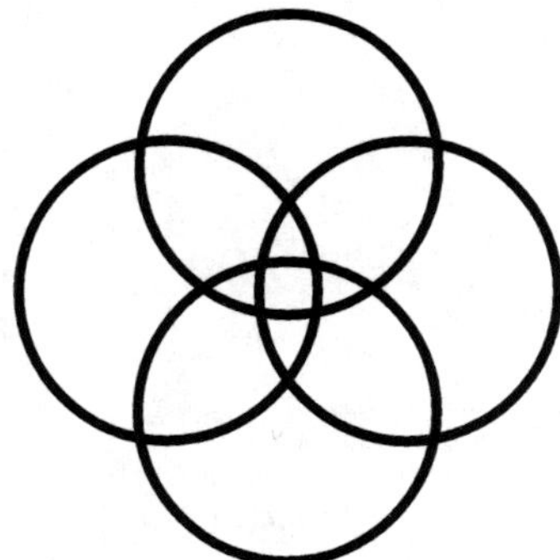

Oxygen Therapy

Question Set 1

1. Based on the information from the nurse on the telephone, what indication do you have that Mr. Feder is potentially hypoxic?

   Elevated heart rate, exacerbation of COPD, physician order

2. What equipment would you bring with you to evaluate, and possibly treat, Mr. Feder?

   Pulse oximeter, nasal cannula, flowmeter, possibly venti-mask

Question Set 2

3. Based on the interview you've just watched, what *observations* did you make about Mr. Feder that indicate potential hypoxia?

   Patient sitting on the edge of the bed in tripod position; pursed-lip breathing; cyanosis of lips; pause during speech to catch breath

4. What is Mr. Feder's chief complaint?

   Increasing dyspnea over the past couple of weeks

5. Describe the history of Mr. Feder's present illness (HPI).

   More trouble catching breath over the past couple of weeks
   Dyspnea at rest
   Trouble concentrating
   Wet cough
   No fever
   No chest pain
   Activities limited
   Dyspnea 5 or 6 on a scale of 1 to 10

6. Describe Mr. Feder's past medical history (PMH).

   Pneumonia 1 year ago
   Smoker—2 PPD x approximately 45 years
   Heart bypass surgery 5 years ago
   Thoracoplasty 50 years ago
   Emphysema x 1 year
   Medicines: inhaler, heart medicine

7. What information from the interview indicates potential hypoxia?

   Increasing dyspnea; dyspnea at rest; trouble concentrating; activities limited; dyspnea 5 to 6 on a scale of 1 to 10; emphysema

8. Based on your facility's policies and procedures, how would you chart this interview?

   Answers will be individualized by institution and should include information from answers to questions 3 through 6.

9. What is a thoracoplasty? For which disease was this procedure commonly performed in the past? If you don't know the answer to these questions, how would you locate this information in your practice setting? Be specific.

   Thoracoplasty is the removal of all or part of one or more ribs, with or without removal of underlying lung. It was formerly used to treat tuberculosis (TB). It reduces the size of the thorax to minimize risk of mediastinal shift when TB reduces lung volume.

   Regarding how RCP would find this out, answers will be specific to institution

10. What additional questions would you ask Mr. Feder?

    Answers will vary; there are many possibilities. Responses should include questions that indicate additional data collection relevant to the interview and hypoxic condition.

Question Set 3

11. A pulse oximeter was used to assess Mr. Feder's oxygenation. What factors indicate a reliable reading from the device, assuming it is properly calibrated?

    Reading stops fluctuating; HR is consistent with pulse or AR; wave form on monitor is consistent; reading makes sense based on clinical presentation.

12. List three patient factors which would make a pulse oximeter reading unreliable.

    Poor perfusion, movement of sensor (tremors), CO poisoning, anemia

13. A different patient you're caring for has a pulse oximeter monitor in place on his fingertip. The patient has a grand mal seizure with tonic-clonic movements. He is grunting, and his lips are cyanotic. Would this affect the pulse oximeter reading? Why or why not? If the reading would be affected, what action would you take?

    Reading would be unreliable because of movement of the sensor. Sensor tip could be replaced with a device that could be clipped on patient's ear lobe.

14. Would a pulse oximeter reading be reliable during a resuscitation? Why or why not?

    Reading would not be reliable because of a lack of peripheral perfusion, as well as motion artifact during external cardiac compressions. Device should not be used.

15. In the space below, chart Mr. Feder's targeted physical examination, based on your facility's policies and procedures.

Specific answers will depend on individual institutions. The following details should be included:
Diminished vesicular breath sounds throughout
Generally decreased tactile fremitus
Generalized increase in resonance
Pulse oximetry reading: 88%
Tachypnea with some respiratory distress
Minimal accessory muscle use
No JVD
No dependent edema

16. Is Mr. Feder hypoxemic or hypoxic? On what data do you base your answer?

Yes, both. This answer is based on pulse oximetry, tachypnea, tachycardia, dyspnea of 5 to 6 on a scale of 1 to 10, cyanosis of lips, and Mr. Feder's trouble concentrating.

17. Based on your assessment data, if you answered yes to the question above, what is the likely cause of Mr. Feder's hypoxemia/hypoxia?

$\dot{V}/\dot{Q}$ mismatch; exacerbation of COPD; no evidence of CHF or infection

18. Review the therapist-driven protocol on page 245. What would your next steps be, based on that algorithm?

Administer oxygen at 2 LPM via nasal cannula.
Monitor pulse oximetry, titrate liter flow to maintain $SpO_2 \geq 92\%$.

Question Set 4

19. List patient teaching points when administering oxygen.

Recognition of why patient is receiving oxygen
Importance of no smoking, as well as being careful with electrical appliances
Importance of wearing oxygen continuously
No open flame

20. How would you assess whether the oxygen being administered is helpful to Mr. Feder?

Pulse oximetry saturation improved; decreased respiratory rate toward normal; decreased heart rate toward normal; decreased dyspnea on 1 to 10 scale; less or absent cyanosis of lips; patient lying more comfortably in bed (no more need of tripod position); patient report of improvement

21. For the blood gas drawn before the patient was admitted to the hospital, write your interpretation.

pH 7.44, $PaCO_2$ 32, PaO_2 52, HCO_3 22, SaO_2 86%
Fully compensated respiratory alklalosis with hypoxemia

22. Based on the arterial blood gas and CBC results, what general statement can you make about Mr. Feder's oxygen-carrying capacity?

Carrying capacity is within normal limits, despite low arterial oxygen tension.

23. If you walked into Mr. Feder's room to reassess him and you collected the following data: HR 110, RR 28, SpO_2 90%, what action would you take, based on the therapist-driven protocol on page 245?

    Increase liter flow on nasal cannula (per TDP)
    Alternative, switch to Venti-mask

24. List three goals of oxygen therapy for Mr. Feder. Include parameters that would indicate these goals were achieved.

    Improve oxygenation (ABG and pulse oximetry)
    Decreased dyspnea (use 1 to 10 scale)
    Reduce cardiac workload (HR, BP)

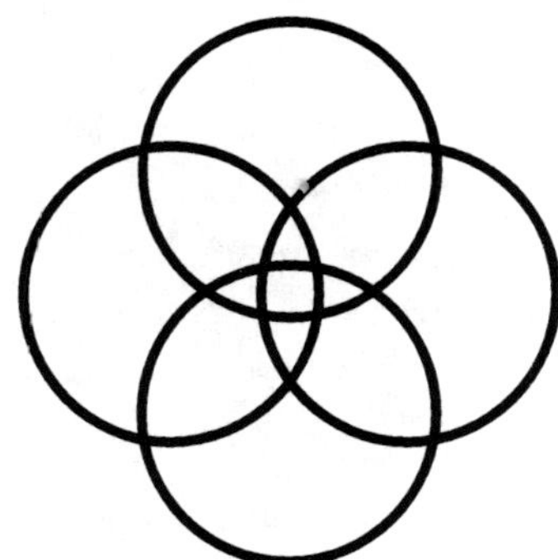

Aerosol Therapy

Question Set 1

1. Based on the information from the nurse on the telephone, what is your initial impression of Mr. Carr?

   Patient admitted with asthma; vitals essentially normal, with slightly elevated HR; anxious, short of breath; asking for treatment

2. Interpret his blood gas results.

   pH 7.51, $PaCO_2$ 29, PaO_2 73, HCO_3 23, SaO_2 94%—room air
   Uncompensated respiratory alkalosis

3. What equipment would you bring to his room?

   Peak flowmeter, pulse oximeter, small-volume nebulizer
   (beta-two agonist liquid and MDI—whether this is brought to the room or obtained on the patient unit depends on hospital policy and procedure)

Question Set 2

4. Based on the interview you just watched, what observations did you make about Mr. Carr's condition?

   Mr. Carr was anxious and fidgety; he used rapid speech and did not need to pause to catch his breath while speaking; his nasal oxygen was at 2 LPM.

5. What is Mr. Carr's chief complaint?

   "My asthma": He woke up at 5 a.m. and couldn't breathe; PEFR in red zone.

6. Describe the history of Mr. Carr's present illness (HPI).

   The day before yesterday, Mr. Carr's peak flow dropped 10%. Yesterday, his peak flow dropped into the yellow zone; this morning at 5 a.m. it was in the red zone. Mr. Carr has new carpeting in his office at work. He has no chest pain.

7. Describe Mr. Carr's past medical history (PMH).

   Diagnosed with asthma on August 23, 1993
   No previous hospitalization
   Occupation: accountant
   Non-smoker
   Eczema
   No accidents or surgery
   Medications: inhaler when PEFR drops; never used PO steroids; take vitamins

8. What other questions might you have asked Mr. Carr?

   Answers will vary; there are many possibilities. Responses should include questions that indicate additional data collection relevant to the interview and asthmatic condition.

9. In the space below, chart this interview, based on your facility's policies and procedures.

   Answers will be individualized by institution and should include information from answers to questions 4 through 7.

Question Set 3

10. In the space below, chart Mr. Carr's targeted physical examination, based on your facility's policies and procedures.

    Format will vary based on institutional policy. The following data should be included:
    Pulse oximetry: SpO_2 96%
    Normal chest excursion
    High-pitched, musical inspiratory and expiratory wheezes throughout all lung fields with prolonged expiratory phase
    PEFR: 50% predicted value

11. How would you describe Mr. Carr's emotional state? How did the RCP in the video address this during the interview and examination?

    Mr. Carr was very anxious.
    RCP refocused his attention back to the interview when he went off on a tangent.
    RCP was very supportive.

12. There were inconsistencies between Mr. Carr's statements and his actions. His statements portray one perspective, yet his actions another. What are some of these inconsistencies? How would you assess his status in the future, taking all factors into account?

    1. He said this was the worst shortness of breath he had ever experienced and rated it 15 on a scale of 1 to 10. Yet, he drove himself to the doctor's office.
    2. He said he couldn't catch his breath, yet he was able to speak in complete sentences without pausing to breathe, and he was able to take slow breaths during auscultation.
    3. He said he used his inhaler every day, even when peak flow was normal.

    Future assessment: use objective data whenever possible—breath sounds, PEFR—to evaluate changes in condition; provide emotional support; point out progress.

13. Describe the pathophysiology which results in Mr. Carr's signs and symptoms.

    Asthma has three components. The primary component is airway inflammation. Additional components are bronchospasm and buildup of thick, tenacious secretions.
    All three contribute to airway obstruction. This airway obstruction is the cause of Mr. Carr's low PEFR, wheezes, dyspnea, and relative hypoxemia.

14. What parameters should you assess to determine the severity of a patient's asthmatic condition? What findings would indicate a worsening in the patient's condition?

    Breath sounds: Assess whether wheezes are present; if so, assess pitch of wheezes (the higher the pitch, the more narrow the airway) and length of expiratory phase (the longer the expiratory phase, the more narrow the airway).

PEFR: Less than 50% predicted is serious.
ABG: Initial hypoxemia not uncommon as a result of $\dot{V}/\dot{Q}$ mismatching. Patient who is tachypneic should have low $PaCO_2$. If $PaCO_2$ is normal with tachypnea, this is a serious sign. If $PaCO_2$ is elevated, this indicates impending respiratory failure.

15. How would you instruct a patient to use a peak flowmeter properly? List the steps of proper use.

    1. Place indicator at base of numerical scale.
    2. Stand up (when possible).
    3. Take a deep breath.
    4. Place meter in mouth with lips closed around the mouthpiece.
    5. Blow out as hard and fast as possible.

    From National Heart, Lung, and Blood Institute: Guidelines for the diagnosis and management of asthma, Bethesda, MD, 1991, Publication Number 91-3042, National Institutes of Health.

16. Mr. Carr is receiving IV Solu-Medrol (methylprednisolone sodium succinate). Why is he receiving this medication? What is its action in treating asthma?

    Solu-Medrol is a corticosteroid, an anti-inflammatory drug. It is used to reduce airway inflammation, which leads to airway obstruction.

17. Review the therapist-driven protocol on page 246. What would your next action be, based on that algorithm?

    Administer bronchodilator therapy via small-volume nebulizer.

Question Set 4

18. How would you assess the effect of the inhaled medication on Mr. Carr?

    Measure peak flow after treatment—look for a significant percentage improvement.
    Assess breath sounds—look for lower-pitched wheezes, more normal expiratory time.
    Assess respiratory rate—look for decreased rate toward normal.
    Assess pulse oximetry—look for normal SpO_2 on room air.
    Assess patient rating of dyspnea on 1 to 10 scale.

19. You return to Mr. Carr's bedside 12 hours later, and your assessment reveals the following: Patient has adequate inspiratory volume; he can hold his breath for 8 seconds; his respiratory rate is 20. How would you proceed, based on the therapist-driven protocol on page 246?

    Administer bronchodilator via metered dose inhaler.

20. List two goals of therapy for Mr. Carr. How will you know when those goals are achieved?

    Improve expiratory airflow—measure PEFR, assess breath sounds.
    Reduce dyspnea—assess respiratory rate, patient report.

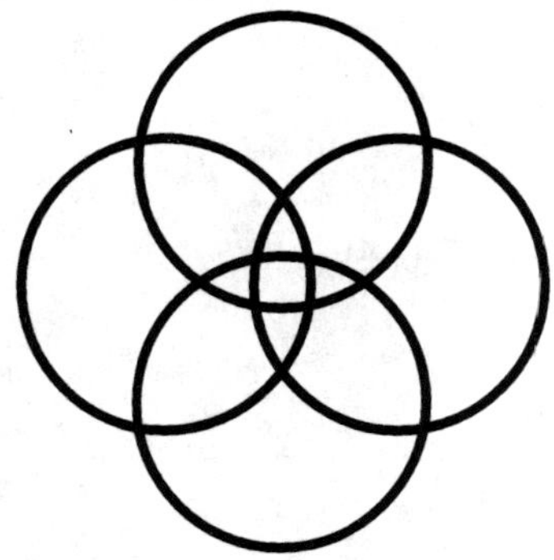

Secretion Management

Question Set 1

1. Based on the information from the nurse on the telephone and your initial chart review, what is Mr. Gonsalves' main problem?

   Lobar pneumonia, right middle lobe

2. What assessment findings are consistent with your answer to question 1?

   Admitting diagnosis, T 104.5, HR 108, RR 32, gram-positive diplococci on sputum gram stain, chest radiograph showing RML pneumonia, hypoxemia on ABG (with hypoventilation consistent with pleuritic pain), elevated WBC on CBC, increased neutrophil count (left shift) consistent with bacterial infection

Question Set 2

3. Based on the interview you just watched, what *observations* did you make about Mr. Gonsalves' condition?

   Tachypnea, grunting with pain, grimacing with pain, appearing ill, IV for hydration, sputum cup with thick yellow sputum at bedside, tissues in emesis basin

4. What is Mr. Gonsalves' chief complaint?

   Pain when he breathes and coughs; trouble getting mucus up; feeling thirsty, "knocked out," and ill: sudden onset of acute illness with pleuritic chest pain

5. Describe the history of Mr. Gonsalves' present illness (HPI).

   Woke up this morning ill; shaking chills and perspiration

6. Describe Mr. Gonsalves' past medical history (PMH).

   Chronic bronchitis
   Usually has productive cough (usually thick white or yellow sputum)
   Inhaler prn
   Smoker—1 1/2 PPD for approximately 30 years

7. What additional questions would you have asked Mr. Gonsalves?

   Suggested responses (RCP may come up with other acceptable answers):
   Is anyone else you know sick? Can you describe your chest pain in more detail: dull, sharp, stabbing? Is the pain related to inspiration? How would you rate the pain on a 1 to 10 scale? What do you do for a living? Have you had a TB test in the last year?

8. In the space below, chart this interview, based on your facility's policies and procedures.

   Answers will be individualized by institution; they should include information from answers to questions 3 through 6.

9. Write your interpretation of Mr. Gonsalves' arterial blood gas results.

   pH 7.32, $PaCO_2$ 56, HCO_3 35, PaO_2 55, SaO_2 86%
   Partially compensated respiratory acidosis with hypoxemia

Question Set 3

10. In the space below, chart Mr. Gonsalves' targeted physical examination, based on your facility's policies and procedures.

    Answers will vary based on institutional policy and should include the following data:
    Pulse oximetry reading: 92%
    Increased tactile fremitus, right middle lobe
    Dull percussion note, right middle lobe
    Breath sounds: vesicular posteriorly, anterior coarse crackles (rhonchi), tubular (or bronchial) sounds right middle lobe, anterior lower chest
    Positive egophony (E to A changes) over right middle lobe

11. During the physical examination, what else did you notice about Mr. Gonsalves' care, consistent with his chief complaint and diagnosis?

    IV for fluid replacement, penicillin G by IV, oxygen by nasal cannula

12. Based on this patient's interview and targeted physical examination, why is Mr. Gonsalves wearing a nasal cannula? Briefly describe the related pathophysiology.

    Nasal cannula is for hypoxemia on initial room-air ABG.
    Pneumonia causes secretions to fill alveoli, causing intrapulmonary shunt and V/Q mismatch.

13. Describe how Mr. Gonsalves' oxygen consumption compares to a normal, healthy person of his same age.

    Increased as a result of increased metabolic demands of fever and increased metabolism fighting acute infection

14. Describe why patients with pneumonia can develop pleuritic chest pain. Describe how patients compensate when they have pleuritic chest pain.

    Pneumonia can irritate adjacent pleural lining. Pleura are highly innervated and, when irritated, cause significant pain. Patients will breathe at smaller tidal volumes and higher rates to minimize lung movement and limit pain.

15. A number of factors can impair normal mucociliary transport. Mr. Gonsalves is experiencing at least five of these factors. List the factors specific to Mr. Gonsalves that are impairing his ability to mobilize secretions.

    Cigarette smoking
    Dehydration
    COPD
    Acute infection—pneumonia
    Medications—narcotic analgesic blunts cough

16. Based on the therapist-driven protocol on page 247, how would you proceed?

    Postural drainage and percussion therapy

17. What additional measures would you take?

    Deep breathing and coughing instruction

Question Set 4

18. Write five contraindications to chest physiotherapy.

    Increased intracranial pressure
    Head and neck injury or surgery
    Uncontrolled airway
    Aspiration risk
    Abnormal coagulation profile
    Bone disease: osteoporosis or recent fracture

19. Write four goals of therapy for Mr. Gonsalves. How would you know if the goals were achieved?

    Increase amount of expectorated sputum—monitor bedside sputum collection cup.
    Reduce abnormal breath sounds—monitor breath sounds for resolution.
    Increase ease in mobilizing secretions—patient report and sputum production.
    Decreased infiltrate on chest radiograph—monitor radiograph results.

20. On follow-up, you note Mr. Gonsalves' breath sounds have changed from bronchial or tubular to coarse crackles. Is this a positive or negative finding? Explain why.

    Positive finding—shows mobilization of sputum

21. Why did the therapist give Mr. Gonsalves his inhaler before his pulmonary hygiene therapy?

    To maximize airway size and, hopefully, to improve secretion mobilization

22. Why did the therapist perform segmental breathing with Mr. Gonsalves?

    To encourage deep breathing in location of RML, since pleuritic pain is causing splinting and limiting inspiratory excursion there

23. Why did the therapist put the pulse oximeter sensor on Mr. Gonsalves during postural drainage?

    To monitor oxygenation and to detect desaturation with position changes

24. How would you continue to monitor Mr. Gonsalves' condition and determine if chest physiotherapy is effective?

    Monitor sputum production with cup at bedside
    Monitor character of sputum
    Monitor breath sounds
    Check chest radiograph results
    Monitor overall condition: vital signs, fever, whether patient continues to feel acutely ill

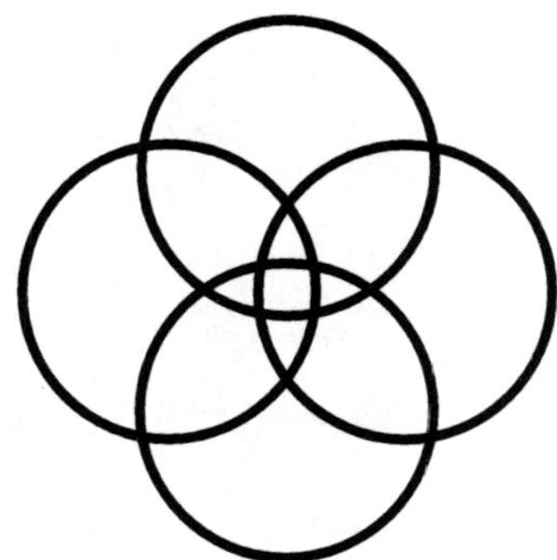

Volume Expansion

Question Set 1

1. Based on the information from the nurse over the telephone, explain why there is an order for respiratory care services for Mrs. Howell.

   75-year-old woman with postop abdominal aortic aneurysm, at risk for postoperative atelectasis and pneumonia due to potential hypoventilation

2. What equipment would you take with you to Mrs. Howell's room?

   Incentive spirometer

Question Set 2

3. Write your interpretation of Mrs. Howell's pre- and postoperative arterial blood gases.

   pH 7.41, $PaCO_2$ 42, HCO_3 28, PaO_2 73, SaO_2 94%—pre-op room air
   ABG normal for age

   pH 7.40, $PaCO_2$ 44, HCO_3 27, PaO_2 62, SaO_2 92%—post-op room air
   ABG normal for age

4. Write your interpretation of Mrs. Howell's vital signs, portable chest radiograph results, and preoperative pulmonary function results.

   All are within normal limits.

5. Based on the interview you just watched, what *observations* did you make about Mrs. Howell's condition?

   Bright, responsive older woman; no obvious distress

6. What is Mrs. Howell's chief complaint?

   Surgery for abdominal aortic aneurysm—worried about incisional pain

7. Describe Mrs. Howell's past medical history (PMH).

   "Female surgery" 25 years ago
   Smoker—1/2 PPD, when younger 1 1/2 PPD for 60 years
   AM "clears throat"; denies cough
   No DOE
   Otherwise negative

8. What other questions might you have asked Mrs. Howell?

   Answers will vary; there are many possibilities. Responses should include questions that indicate additional data collection relevant to the interview and postoperative condition.

9. In the space below, chart this interview, based on your facility's policies and procedures.

   Answers will be individualized by institution and should include information from answers to questions 5 through 7.

Question Set 3

10. In the space below, chart Mrs. Howell's targeted physical examination, based on your facility's policies and procedures.

    Format will vary based on institutional policy. The following data should be included:
    Moderately decreased tactile fremitus
    Normal percussion resonance
    Normal vesicular breath sounds, decreased aeration at bases—improved when patient encouraged to take in deep breath

11. How does treatment of postoperative pain affect a patient's respiratory status?

    Narcotic analgesics blunt the cough reflex and depress respirations.
    Sigh reflex is depressed.
    Epidural analgesia and patient-controlled analgesia reduce central effects and provide better pain relief with fewer effects on respiration.

12. What is a sigh, and how is the normal sigh mechanism affected postoperatively? Why is this important?

    A sigh is an involuntary, slow, deep breath followed by end-inspiratory pause.
    Sighs open collapsed alveoli by increasing transpulmonary pressure.
    General anesthesia effects, narcotic analgesics, and splinting from pain all reduce the depth and frequency of normal sigh breaths. This can lead to underventilated alveoli, regional hypoventilation, and atelectasis.

13. What factors in Mrs. Howell's case will increase pulmonary secretions? How might this complicate her recovery?

    Smoking
    Intubation for general anesthesia causes tracheal irritation, stimulating secretions.
    Inhalation anesthetics cause tracheal irritation, stimulating secretions.

    Increased volume of secretions are harder to clear. Mrs. Howell is afraid to cough because of incisional pain. This situation puts her at risk for retained secretions and postoperative pneumonia.

14. Why is Mrs. Howell at risk for decreased thoracic expansion? How might this complicate her recovery?

    Splinting due to incisional pain
    Abdominal binder
    Depressed respiratory effort from narcotic analgesics and residual anesthesia

    All may lead to shallow breathing, which can lead to atelectasis.

15. Intermittent positive pressure breathing and incentive spirometry are both devices used to enhance deep breathing postoperatively. Compare and contrast how these devices accomplish this therapeutic goal.

    IPPB uses positive pressure to push air into the patient's lung. An increased transpulmonary pressure gradient is created by the positive pressure within the alveoli, which, theoretically, allows deeper breaths.

    Incentive spirometry creates a similar transpulmonary pressure gradient but accomplishes this by creating a higher negative intrathoracic pressure when the patient uses the device to take in deep breaths.

    Incentive spirometry can be performed independently by the patient after initial instruction. IPPB is administered by the RCP.

16. Based on the assessment you've watched and the therapist-driven protocol on page 248, as well as the additional information that Mrs. Howell is able to achieve 80% of her predicted inspiratory capacity, what therapy is appropriate for Mrs. Howell?

    Incentive spirometry

Question Set 4

17. Why is it important to consider a psychosocial assessment when administering incentive spirometry therapy?

    A psychosocial assessment will provide clues as to whether the patient is likely to perform the sustained maximal inspiration maneuver independently every hour, as recommended.

18. Write two goals of therapy for Mrs. Howell. How will you know if these goals are achieved?

    Improvement in diminished breath sounds, evidenced by auscultation
    Absence of atelectasis, evidenced by physical examination and chest radiograph
    Daily increase in inspiratory capacity, evidenced by improved performance with incentive spirometer

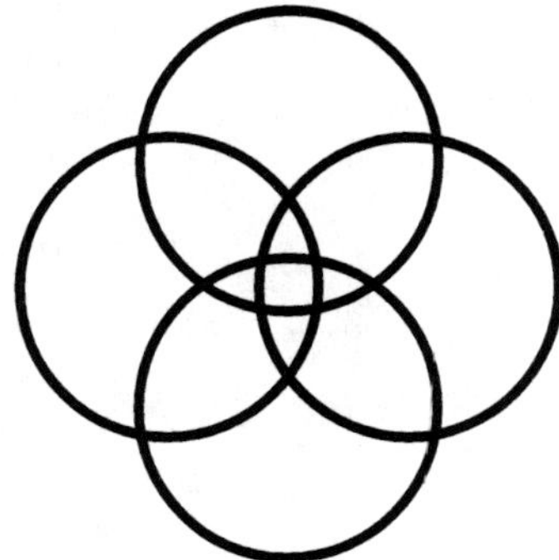

Physical Assessment

Question Set 1

1. Simply by standing at the patient's bedside, what clues do you have from this scene that help you assess the patient's airway and breathing?

   The nurse's report says the patient is complaining of shortness of breath—if he can speak, he has a patent airway and is breathing spontaneously.
   Patient is moaning.
   Patient's breathing can be heard—no stridor or other sounds of obstruction.

2. Interpret the patient's vital signs.

   HR 124, RR 24, BP 90/62
   Tachycardia, tachypnea, borderline hypotension
   Would expect blood pressure to be higher in patient in pain
   May be bleeding into fractured femur or chest

3. Based on the nurse's description alone, what do you think could account for Mr. Donovan's complaints of chest pain and shortness of breath?

   Answers could include almost anything relevant in trauma setting. Potential answers include the following:
   Rib fractures
   Referred pain from arm fracture
   Pneumothorax/hemothorax
   Dissecting aorta/aortic tear
   Cardiac contusion
   Pericardial tamponade

Question Set 2

4. So what do you think? How would you answer the nurse's question?

   Mr. Donovan has slightly decreased breath sounds, slightly increased resonance to percussion, decreased chest wall movement, and significant pain on palpation—all at anterior upper left chest (same side as possible arm fracture).
   May have fractured ribs, which would account for pain and splinting
   May have fractured ribs and pneumothorax, which would also explain slight increased resonance to percussion
   SpO_2 improved with supplemental oxygen

5. Why was Mr. Donovan given oxygen by nonrebreather mask?

   SpO_2 on room air: 88%
   Setting of trauma, possible chest trauma, chest injury
   Patient breathing spontaneously
   Need to administer as much oxygen as possible while completing assessment to reduce risk for hypoxemia and subsequent tissue hypoxia

6. Describe the findings of the inspection portion of Mr. Donovan's exam.

   No cyanosis
   No facial swelling or evidence of facial trauma
   No bruising or evidence of external or penetrating injury to anterior chest wall
   Decreased expansion on left side of chest with inspiration

7. Two elements of inspection in Mr. Donovan's exam were not performed. What was eliminated, why was it not done, and what are the implications for future monitoring and assessment?

   Mr. Donovan's neck was not inspected for tracheal position/deviation and evaluation of neck vein distension. This was not done because the cervical collar blocked the assessment. If the rest of the assessment pointed to a significant pneumothorax or potential cardiac tamponade, the assessment would be very important, and the collar would need to be removed while another professional maintained c-spine immobilization. Otherwise, the assessment can be postponed for now, while the potential neck injury is being evaluated first.

   His back was also not inspected. Because of the risk of further injury to Mr. Donovan's neck by moving him, this inspection can be postponed. His other assessment findings are all consistent, and his condition is stable, so this assessment can be postponed—unless his condition changes.

8. After inspection, the RCP squeezed Mr. Donovan's finger. What is the significance of this maneuver?

   The RCP was checking capillary refill. When the nailbed is compressed, it will turn white. When it is released, it should return to the normal pink color within two seconds.
   This is a rudimentary assessment of perfusion.
   Mr. Donovan's capillary refill was normal.

9. List three different assessments that are done when palpating a trauma patient's chest.

   Skin temperature and moisture (warm, cold, clammy, dry, diaphoretic)
   Stability of thoracic cage, bony structures
   Areas of localized pain or tenderness
   Crepitus or subcutaneous emphysema

10. What is the significance of Mr. Donovan's percussion findings in the setting of chest trauma?

    Findings could indicate pneumothorax due to slightly increased resonance.
    Findings do not support bleeding in chest, which would result in dull percussion.

11. Write your interpretation of Mr. Donovan's heart and lung sounds.

    Heart: normal sounds, tachycardia
    Lungs: Normal vesicular sounds with somewhat decreased aeration (sounds), left upper anterior chest

12. Why is an assessment of circulation important in a trauma patient?

    The circulatory system carries the oxygen-rich blood to the tissues. If the patient is in shock, or if circulation is decreased, oxygen may not be delivered to the tissues. Tissue hypoxia as a result of circulatory hypoxia can occur.

13. What factors put Mr. Donovan at risk for airway obstruction or aspiration?

    Cervical spine immobilization—forced supine position
    Intoxication—more likely to vomit
    Potential for head injury
    Potential for decreased level of consciousness
    Potential for soft-tissue swelling

14. What should be done next?

    Place patient on monitor for continuous EKG and pulse oximetry monitoring.
    Chest radiograph
    Cervical spine radiograph
    ABG
    Other studies as needed (may include a variety of responses)

15. In the space below, chart this assessment, using your facility's policies and procedures.

    Answers will be individualized by institution; they should include information from answers to questions 4, 6, and 11.

Question Set 3

16. Interpret Mr. Donovan's ABG results.

    pH 7.41 $PaCO_2$ 34, HCO_3 21, PO_2 317, SaO_2 99%
    Essentially normal, or fully compensated, respiratory alklalosis with hyperoxia

17. What are Mr. Donovan's vital signs now? How do you interpret these findings?

    HR 85, sinus rhythm, RR 26, SpO_2 98%, BP 122/93
    Vital signs within normal limits following chest-tube placement; RR still elevated; probably has reduced tidal volume as a result of splinting on left side.
    Respiratory rate increases to maintain minute volume; RR could be also be increased because of pain.

18. On the first radiograph, there are three solid circles and a D-shaped ring in bright white on the film. What do these represent?

    The circles are the EKG leads, with wires attached.
    The ring is from the sling for the broken arm.

19. When the RCP looked at the chest drain, there was bubbling in the middle chamber when Mr. Donovan coughed, as well as continuous bubbling in the left chamber. What do these chambers and findings represent?

    The middle chamber is the water seal. Bubbling with coughing indicates air leaking from the lung. The left chamber is the suction control. Continuous bubbling indicates that excess negativity from the suction source is being vented to the atmosphere—and that the amount of negative pressure applied to the pleural space is equal to the level of water in this chamber.

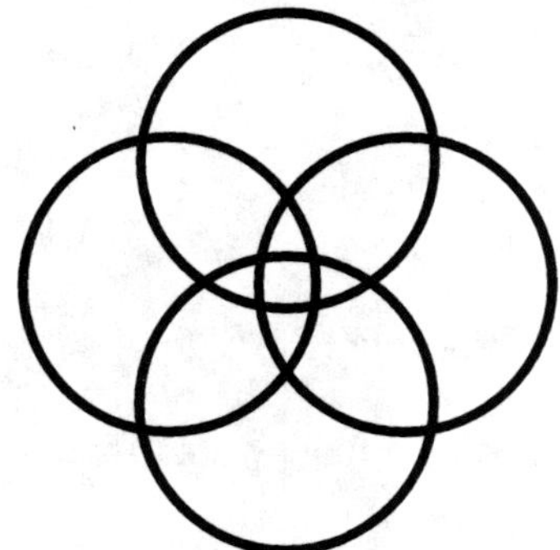

Pediatrics

Question Set 1

1. Based on the interview you just watched, what *observations* did you make about Alyssa's condition?

   Shy, not talking
   Acyanotic
   No obvious respiratory distress

2. What is Alyssa's chief complaint?

   "Nasty, barking cough"

3. Describe the history of Alyssa's present illness (HPI).

   Didn't feel good after daycare, has had runny nose past couple of days, didn't eat much at dinner, went to bed early, woke up with barking cough
   No fever, no sore throat or drooling, is able to drink fluids

4. Describe Alyssa's past medical history (PMH).

   Typical colds and ear infections of childhood; immunizations up to date

5. What do you think is responsible for Alyssa's condition?

   Viral upper airway infection—croup

Question Set 2

6. What is the significance of the pulse oximetry assessment in this case?

   Pulse oximetry was normal. If airway obstruction were severe, SpO_2 could drop, indicating a need for supplemental oxygen and possible impending respiratory failure.

7. When the RCP tried to listen to Alyssa's lungs, she became fussy and pulled away. He decided to defer the assessment. Do you agree or disagree with his action? Explain your rationale.

   Based on this history, the site of the infection is likely the upper airway, not the lungs. Auscultation of stridor confirms this. There is no evidence of bronchitis or pneumonia. Her fussiness can increase her metabolic demands, increase her respiratory rate, and worsen the upper airway obstruction. Fighting with her and insisting on listening to her lungs may have worsened her condition. If a child is crying, it is very difficult to assess the lungs with the vocalization, anyway. The RCP could check with the physician or nurse to see if they were able to listen to her lungs while she was quiet.

8. What would you recommend for Alyssa's treatment?

   Racemic epinephrine aerosol to reduce airway edema

9. In the space below, chart this assessment, using your facility's policies and procedures.

   Answers will be individualized by institution; they should include information from answers to questions 1 through 4.

Question Set 3

10. Interpret Alyssa's vital signs.

    T 100.2 tympanic, BP 90/60, HR 120, RR 32
    Essentially normal for age, with slightly elevated HR and RR, consistent with upper airway obstruction. No evidence of severe distress

11. On the physician's order sheet, along with an order for racemic epinephrine, is an order for prednisolone oral solution. What is the therapeutic effect of this drug? Why is it prescribed for Alyssa? If you do not know the answer to these questions, what resources in your institution would you use to get information about the drug? Be specific.

    It is a corticosteroid, anti-inflammatory drug used in croup to reduce airway edema.
    Answer to resources will be individualized by institution.

12. Based on your facility's policies and procedures, how would you prepare to administer the racemic epinephrine to Alyssa?

    Answer will be individualized by institution. It should include equipment used and diluent solution and volume.

Question Set 4

13. When the RCP returned to the bedside, he brought a teddy bear and an extra equipment set-up. Why did he do this?

    Alyssa is a preschooler. Children in this age group are particularly afraid of body mutilation, darkness, and loss of control. Preschool children work through their anxieties and fears with play.
    By administering a "pretend" treatment to the teddy bear, using the very same equipment that will be used on Alyssa, the RCP gives her a chance to play with the equipment and become familiar with it. Ideally, this will make the actual treatment less frightening to Alyssa.

14. If you were having a problem working with a child in your institution, what resources could you contact for assistance?

    Answer will be individualized by institution. Child life specialists are specially trained professionals who help children cope with the fears and anxieties associated with health care and medical treatments and procedures. Many hospitals have child life centers. Other resources might include parents and other pediatric staff such as nurses.

15. Many hospitals have special policies regarding disposition of children following racemic epinephrine treatments for upper airway obstruction. Why are special policies sometimes implemented? What is the policy in your institution?

    Rebound edema with subsequent airway obstruction can occur after racemic epinephrine via aerosol. Some institutions require admission for observation if a racemic epinephrine treatment is given. Other institutions allow discharge if oral steroids have been given, the caregiver is reliable, there is quick access to care if the child's condition deteriorates at home, and the child is monitored for two to three hours in the ED before discharge.
    Answers regarding institutional policy will vary.

16. Write a goal of therapy for Alyssa.

    Reduce airway obstruction

17. How will you assess the results of the treatment to determine if your goal is met?

    Auscultate neck for stridor; assess respiratory rate, color

Question Set 5

18. What are the results of the racemic epinephrine treatment given to Alyssa? What would you recommend at this point?

    Stridor is gone. Child is sleeping, in no distress.
    Suggest observation in ED one or two more hours. If no further evidence of obstruction and child is able to drink without difficulty, discharge.

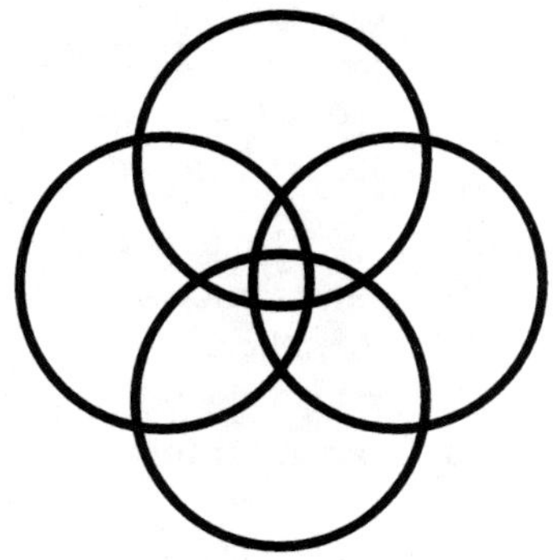

Noninvasive Monitoring

Question Set 1

1. Based on the discussion with the nurse alone, what noninvasive monitoring tools would you recommend be used for this patient?

   EKG, noninvasive blood pressure, pulse oximetry, capnometry

2. Interpret Ms. Reilly's blood gases.

   pH 7.37, $PaCO_2$ 41, PaO_2 148, SaO_2 99%
   Essentially normal readings

3. What is gastric lavage? Why is it done? If you don't know the answer to this question, what resources in your institution would you use to acquire the information? Be specific.

   Gastric lavage consists of placing a large tube through the mouth into the stomach. Fluid is injected into the tube with an irrigating syringe, and then the fluid is withdrawn. This procedure is primarily used to remove toxic substances, such as pill fragments, from the stomach following overdose. The answer concerning resources for this information will vary based on institution.

4. Why are some patients intubated before gastric lavage?

   If a patient has a decreased level of consciousness as a result of drug overdose, the cough reflex may be blunted. If the cough reflex is blunted, the patient may not be able to protect the airway from foreign substances. During lavage, patients sometimes vomit around the irrigation tube. Aspiration can result. A cuffed endotracheal tube allows the patient to be ventilated and to receive oxygen, while protecting the airway from aspiration injury.

5. The nurse stated that the treatment for a widened QRS complex in tricyclic overdose is serum alkalinization. How can this be accomplished with mechanical ventilation?

   Intentional hyperventilation with mechanical ventilation will lower $PaCO_2$ values. As $PaCO_2$ values drop, pH will rise. This will accomplish serum alkalinization without administration of sodium bicarbonate.

Question Set 2

6. An assessment of intubated patients that should be done at least once per shift was not illustrated here. What is it, and how would you perform this assessment?

   The cuff inflation should be assessed. After suctioning through the patient's mouth above the cuff—and while another professional manually ventilates the patient with a manual resuscitation bag—the RCP should listen to the patient's neck for a minimal leak with positive pressure ventilation. If a minimal leak is not heard, air should be withdrawn or added to the cuff until this is accomplished. The cuff pressure should then be measured.

7. Why did the RCP look where the endotracheal tube was taped at the mouth corner?

   The length marking at the mouth corner should be noted at least once per shift (or more often, depending on institutional policy). If a subsequent assessment reveals a different marking at the mouth corner, this provides evidence that the tube has moved. Proper intervention can then be undertaken.

8. The RCP looked at the distal end of the T-tube reservoir tubing. Why did he do this? If no mist can be seen, what should be done?

   The RCP looks to see if mist is still present at peak inspiration. A disappearing mist indicates the patient's peak inspiratory flow is greater than the output of the system. The total system flow should be increased. Institutional policy and procedure will determine how this is done.

9. In the space below, chart this assessment, based on your facility's policies and procedures.

   Format will vary based on institutional policy. The following data should be included:
   Breath sounds: clear vesicular, equal bilaterally
   ET tube with 23 cm at mouth corner
   EKG: sinus tachycardia 140
   Patient unresponsive to voice
   ABG normal
   T-tube 40%, mist seen at peak inspiration

Question Set 3

10. Pulse oximetry was used to monitor Ms. Reilly's condition. Give five factors that will affect the readings or limit the precision or performance of this device.

    Motion artifact
    Abnormal hemoglobin, such as carboxyhemoglobin and methemoglobin
    Intravascular dyes
    Ambient light on the sensor
    Low perfusion
    Skin pigmentation
    Nail covering (artificial nails) with finger probe
    Saturation below 83%

11. What is the primary reason to use capnography to monitor Ms. Reilly?

    To detect hypoventilation from respiratory depression as a result of the overdose

12. What are four other clinical uses of capnography?

    To detect inadvertent esophageal intubation immediately following placement of endotracheal tube
    To detect leaks around endotracheal tube cuff during mechanical ventilation
    As a monitor during weaning to determine the patient's ability to resume the work of breathing
    To monitor return of diaphragmatic function in patients receiving neuromuscular blocking drugs
    In detecting pulmonary embolic events when monitoring $P(a\text{-}et)CO_2$

Question Set 4

13. Using the pulse oximetry protocol on page 250, how would you answer the nurse's question? Can pulse oximetry be discontinued?

    Yes. The patient's condition is stable without supplemental oxygen, with normal saturation on room air.

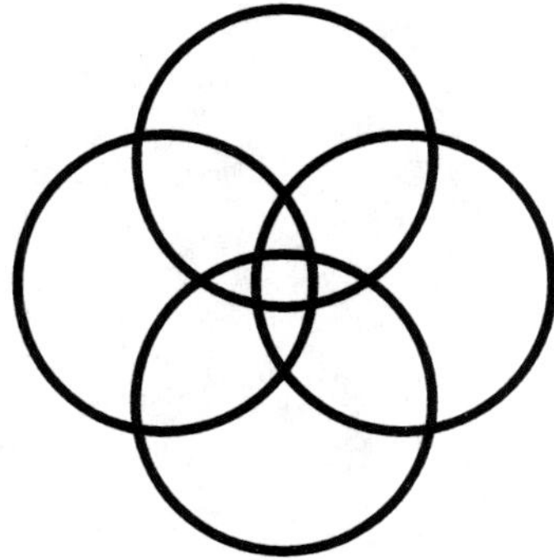

Mechanical Ventilation

Question Set 1

1. Interpret Mrs. Gleason's blood gases.

   pH 7.43, $PaCO_2$ 37, PaO_2 98, SaO_2 97%
   Normal; PaO_2 lower than expected on 40% oxygen

2. What will you need to monitor for, based on the report you just heard?

   Neurological status (When patient wakes up, evaluate for weaning.)
   Congestive heart failure as a result of MI with pulmonary edema

Question Set 2

3. Using the ventilator flow sheet on page 252, compare the current findings to those of the last ventilator check.
   Peak pressure is higher.
   Compliance is lower.
   Breath sounds now have crackles in bases.
   HR is increased.
   SpO_2 is decreased.

Question Set 3

4. In the space below, chart Mrs. Gleason's assessment, based on your facility's policies and procedures.

   Format will vary based on institutional policy. The following data should be included:
   Answer to question 3
   Breath sounds with crackles throughout dependent, posterior lung fields
   Low urine output

5. Describe the pathophysiology responsible for the clinical signs now evident in Mrs. Gleason.

   The myocardial infarction damages myocardial tissue. If enough muscle tissue is damaged, the heart's pumping action will be affected. If the heart cannot pump effectively, blood will back up in the system, first in the left ventricle, then in the left atrium, and next, in the pulmonary circulation. If blood backs up in the pulmonary circulation, hydrostatic pressure will exceed oncotic pressure, and fluid will spill out into the interstitial space and alveoli. This results in pulmonary edema and the clinical signs evident in Mrs. Gleason.

6. Interpret Mrs. Gleason's most recent ABG.

   7.41, $PaCO_2$ 42, PaO_2 70, SaO_2 92%
   Normal, with relative hypoxia on 40% oxygen

Normal, with relative hypoxia on 40% oxygen

7. Review the therapist-driven protocol of mechanical ventilation on page 251. Based on the protocol, what should the RCP do next? Do you agree or disagree with this recommendation? What is your rationale?

   The protocol indicates the next step would be to increase FIO_2. However, the pathophysiology for this condition is pulmonary edema, which produces a shunt effect. Increasing FIO_2 is likely to have little effect on oxygenation.

8. What would you recommend as the next intervention for Mrs. Gleason? What is your rationale?

   Add PEEP to treat shunt. PEEP will, ideally, increase the volume of the alveoli and thus decrease the fluid/volume ratio. PEEP may also redistribute lung water to other areas and reopen collapsed or obstructed respiratory bronchioles, allowing air to flow more freely. Ideally, all these factors work together to improve ventilation/perfusion matching, reduce shunting, and improve oxygenation.

Question Set 4

9. Vaun, Mrs. Gleason's nurse, administered these medications: nitroglycerin, digitalis, and furosemide. What categories do each of these drugs fall into, and why are they being given to Mrs. Gleason? If you don't know the answer, what resources would you use in your institution to acquire this information? Be specific.

   Nitroglycerin (vasodilator): Increases coronary blood flow, decreases systemic vascular resistance, or afterload. There will be less resistance for the heart to pump against, and, theoretically, cardiac output will rise.
   Digitalis (cardiac glycoside): Increases contractility—pumping action of the heart.
   Strengthens cardiac contraction. Theoretically, increases cardiac output.
   For both of these drugs, more effective pumping of the heart will decrease the backup of blood in the pulmonary circulation and will reduce pulmonary edema.
   Furosemide (diuretic): Increases urine output. This will decrease intravascular fluid overload and, theoretically, reduce pulmonary edema.

10. How will you monitor Mrs. Gleason's condition to determine if interventions are having the desired effect?

    Measure peak and plateau pressures; calculate compliance
    Assess oxygenation with pulse oximetry and ABG
    Assess breath sounds for decreased crackles
    Evaluate urine for increased output

Question Set 5

11. Based on the changes in Mrs. Gleason's status, what would you recommend next?

    Continue to monitor, now that Mrs. Gleason is awake; measure weaning parameters to assess readiness to begin weaning.

Notes

Notes

Notes

Notes

Notes

Notes

Notes

Notes

Notes

Notes

Notes